THE
UNKINDEST
CUT

THE
UNKINDEST
CUT

LIFE IN
THE BACKROOMS
OF MEDICINE

MARCIA MILLMAN

William Morrow and Company, Inc.
New York   1977

Printed in the United States of America.

2   3   4   5   6   7   8   9   10

Library of Congress Cataloging in Publication Data

Millman, Marcia.
   The unkindest cut.

   Bibliography: p.
      1. Hospitals—Medical staff.   2. Hospitals—Sociological aspects.   3. Hospital care.   4. Physicians—Discipline. 5. Surgeons.   I. Title. [DNLM: 1. Hospital medical staff— Popular works.   2. Surgery—Popular works.   3. Quality of health care—Popular works.
   WB50.1 M655u]
   RA972.M48   1977   362.1'1   76-18726
   ISBN 0-688-03120-X

BOOK DESIGN   CARL WEISS

For

ESTHER SCHRAGER MILLMAN

and for

HARRY MILLMAN

CONTENTS

PART III/ OTHER BACKROOMS OF MEDICINE

INTRODUCTION

THIS BOOK OFFERS a description and analysis of some of
the "backrooms" of American medicine: a look at what is
said and done in operating rooms, at Mortality Review Conferences, in the Emergency Room, and at various kinds of
hospital staff meetings. The focus of the book is on features
of the everyday world of the hospital that adversely affect
the quality of patient care.

The situations and events described in this book are ones
I personally observed during a two-year-long sociological
study of doctors and staff at work in a private, university-
affiliated hospital. In reporting my observations I have
changed only the names and a few identifying features of
individuals; otherwise, my descriptions are based entirely
upon actual incidents. As a sociologist interested in problems of health care, I was given permission by hospital administrators, department chiefs and research committees to
attend and observe the daily events on the hospital wards, in
the operating rooms, at teaching rounds, and at various staff
conferences.

At first, my research interests were quite general. I soon
found, however, that my attentions were drawn toward two
intriguing issues. One was the variety of ways that doctors
define, perceive and respond to medical mistakes—both their
own mistakes and those made by hospital colleagues. In
particular, I became interested in the ways that doctors
systematically ignore and justify medical errors, or treat them
as if they are inconsequential. What interested me about
medical mistakes was not the fact that they occur, for as

the saying goes, everyone makes mistakes. Nor was I especially interested in the fact that they occur with great frequency, since by now that is fairly common knowledge. Rather, I was interested in the fact that when they *do* occur, they are perpetuated and ignored by physician-colleagues, and furthermore, that this response is built into the organization of hospital life and the professional training and outlook of physicians. As I demonstrate through case studies, the lines of authority and responsibility, even in teaching hospitals, are often sufficiently ambiguous to allow for a pervasive lack of control in matters of incompetence, the exercise of "poor judgment" (as physicians like to call it) and serious errors.

In addition to organizational laxity about physician regulation, doctors share many justifications and excuses for making mistakes and for not pointing out each other's incompetence or poor judgment. These justifications are learned in professional training and are supported in the daily practice of medical work. Rationalizations for mistakes and for not criticizing colleagues are encouraged by the familiar medical claim that each case is "unique." Physicians are reluctant to specify agreed upon treatments for standardly measured indications of illness. Instead they defend the importance of personal experience and "clinical judgment." Indeed, doctors argue that medicine is an "art" rather than a science. And naturally, it is much more difficult for physician-peers to criticize and evaluate each other's "artistic" judgments and performances than it would be for them to hold each other responsible for conforming to standard practices in objectively measured situations. The consequence is that physicians are not held accountable for what they do. Furthermore, as I illustrate through several case studies, physicians come to view their patients in ways that allow them to blame the patient-victims for what are actually medical errors.

These professionally sanctioned justifications and excuses for mistakes are ritualized in institutional ceremonies such as the Medical Mortality Review Conferences. For, as I describe in the book, although the avowed purpose of these meetings is to investigate possible physician errors, in actual practice these meetings typically serve to relieve doctors from feeling responsible for a patient's death.

The study of mistakes affords a good opportunity to observe how members of work groups support each other in sustaining views they would like to hold of themselves, for mistakes often threaten these views. The study of mistakes in medicine is especially interesting, for here the stakes are so high and the consequences so serious that the process of justifying mistakes takes a central place in the life of the work and the profession.

The second major issue I came to focus on is the competing interests and conflicts among various groups of doctors within the hospital. The hospital staff of a private teaching hospital is composed of three different groups of doctors that have conflicting interests. First, there are private, "attending" physicians who admit their patients to the hospital; second, there are house officers (or housestaff): residents and interns receiving their clinical training while they provide hospital service; third, there are full-time, senior staff members who work either in a teaching or supervisory position (such as chief of a department) or a service capacity (such as an anesthesiologist or pathologist).

Clashes among the groups often get expressed over the care of specific patients or over hospital policies. Patients are frequently the ultimate victims of these conflicts, which are built into the organization of hospital work. For example, residents and interns tend to regard their work as an opportunity to learn about "interesting" or esoteric diseases. They are chronically annoyed with private attending doctors who bring to the hospital patients suffering from commonplace illnesses. The residents feel that caring for patients with chronic diseases is a waste of their time and talents, and an abuse of their services. While the private doctors can at least collect fees for daily hospital visits, these patients mean only additional unpleasant work for the housestaff. As I illustrate, the house officers' resentment frequently gets expressed in the care they give to these patients.

In addition to examining the tensions between these groups of doctors, I also examine the conflicts between various departments of the hospital. For example, anesthesiologists and surgeons often struggle over control of the operating room and the Intensive Care Unit. And cardiologists (who are medical specialists) and cardiac surgeons often argue over the appropriate treatment for patients with heart disease. Although American physicians tend to congratulate themselves for their disagreements, and maintain that these disputes contribute to a high quality of medical care, I illustrate how these conflicts often result in activities that endanger the lives and welfare of patients.

The conflicts are important not only because of their frequency and consequences but because they reflect important political and economic changes taking place in the organization of American medical care. In the growing conflict between the "organization" of medicine (as represented by senior full-time staff and house officers) and attending physicians in private practice, we see at the local level of the hospital a reproduction of struggles taking place on a national level. Technological developments in medicine have contributed to a decline in "solo practice," and physicians are increasingly dependent on hospitals and other organizations for carrying out their work. These changes have threatened the traditional autonomy of physicians in private practice and their conflicts with other groups in the hospital reflect these trends.

Throughout the book I try to demonstrate how the practical interests and realities of the physicians' work lives shape the way they look at the world and at patients and illness. I show how the physicians' perspectives serve to protect their own interests rather than those of patients. For even with the best of intentions, most doctors come to see things in ways that make their work easier or more profitable. Although many of the situations I describe are extremely disturbing, I wish to emphasize that they are not created by sinister intentions of individual physicians, but rather are allowed and fostered by structural features of professional and hospital organization. Many of the physicians described in this book were hard-working, well-meaning individuals. Some were disturbed by the things they observed happening around them in the hospital, although few took any action to make changes. Doctors are probably no different or worse than members of any other group in their fallibility and desire to ignore or hide mistakes, or in paying more attention to their personal concerns than those of their clients. But because of their unusual power and privilege in this society, and the special nature of their work, doctors' beliefs and behavior are rarely challenged. Their activities are remarkably free from any control or regulation, and they are seldom held accountable for their performances. And of course, their mistakes and self-serving tendencies are more directly consequential than those of most other individuals.

The reader may wonder whether the incidents I describe are typical or unusual. My own research and that of others indicate that the situations I have portrayed are commonly found in American hospitals. In fact, this book describes a much better than average group of physicians who work at a prestigious institution where they encounter more regulation (though it is disturbingly scant) than physicians at non-teaching hospitals. On the other hand, although I tried to be fair, I did not write extensively about the many "good" things that I observed doctors do, for I was interested in calling attention to the problems I saw. The doctors and incidents I describe, then, should be viewed as neither the best nor the worst of American medicine. More precisely, I have described some of the worst things commonly done even by some of the best doctors. I have portrayed the disturbing things frequently occurring even in the health care offered to relatively wealthy and knowledgeable patients in highly regarded institutions. The reader may safely assume that the care offered to the poor, or to individuals in rural areas, is considerably worse.

My usual method in this research was to attach myself for a time to a particular physician (most often a resident, but frequently a department chief or an attending doctor) and to follow that individual throughout his or her daily rounds of the hospital. For example, on the days I followed a surgical resident or team of residents I would arrive at the hospital at six-thirty in the morning, change into a surgical dress and laboratory coat, and accompany my residents first on morning rounds, then to breakfast, and afterward into the operating room where they would spend a large part of the day. During surgery I usually stationed myself next to the anesthesiologist, by the patient's shoulders, so that I could watch the operation and listen to the conversations of the surgeons and staff as they worked. Between operations I joined the residents and nurses in the operating room (OR) staff lounge, so that I could learn what was happening in other operating suites. Since I was free to wander I could then circulate to whatever operating rooms were the scenes of interesting incidents on any particular day.

After surgery, I joined the residents as they made afternoon rounds throughout the wards, performed "work-up" examinations, and attended various staff meetings. On patient rounds, when I was introduced at all, it was simply as "Dr. Millman" and "one of the team." I ate lunch and dinner with the residents I followed. Occasionally, when the resident I followed was on night call, I, too, stayed in the hospital through the night.

By spending so much time with individuals and by accompanying them through their entire days for weeks or months at a time I was able to get a feeling for the texture and quality of staff life in the hospital. I was able to observe how the various groups of doctors viewed and gave meaning to the situations which arose, and how they chose to pay attention to some things and not to others. Because I was present for such a long time, I was able not only to observe their behavior, but I could also ask physicians about their thoughts and feelings in the course of ongoing events. I kept careful notes of my observations, and stopped several times a day to write detailed descriptions of conversations and incidents.

In addition to following individuals through their rounds of work, I collected other information systematically. For example, I attended all the Medical Mortality Review Conferences held during the period of my research, and I attended many of the daily "Chief's Reports" meetings between the residents and the Chief of Medicine. At times, instead of following one individual throughout the day, I would station myself permanently at particular locations in the hospital that seemed important to understand in their own right. Thus, I spent a few months observing activities in the Emergency Room, and a few more following the events on one combined medical-surgical patient ward.

In addition to my informal conversations during the course of a day, I conducted more formal, extended interviews with various department chiefs, staff members and attending physicians and administrators. I explained to all of them that I was studying the things that came up routinely in their work. With most I discussed my particular interest in understanding the conflicts between different groups within the hospital and in the behavior surrounding physicians' mistakes. Although some of the doctors were uneasy about being observed, they were by and large surprisingly friendly, generous, and cooperative in allowing me to join them in their world. Some even went to considerable trouble to make sure that I felt "included" or that I understood all the implications and background of what I saw. A few became my special allies and "sociological" collaborators. They seemed to enjoy the opportunity to step out of their usual perspective and view their work and behavior as a sociologist would.

Since the long-term nature of my research allowed me to construct friendly relations with some of the physicians, I observed and talked with them not only in work situations and in formal interviews, but also at parties, over coffee, in staff lounges, and at dinner in their homes. The style and intensity of this method of research allowed me to gather the kind of information and understanding I wanted: I followed doctors closely enough to share some of their experiences, or at least to see them firsthand, yet since I was a sociologist-observer rather than one of their group, I could maintain an independent perspective on what I saw.

One might wonder how it is possible to spend day after day with people, to know them over long periods of time, even to pay friendly visits to their homes, all the while seeing them as subjects of research and their lives as sociological data. In fact, the complexities of this problem are often the subjects of long conversations among sociologists who do this kind of "participant-observation" research, and a few important considerations can be identified.

Learning to be an effective participant-observer generally involves an extensive training and learning process. The observer learns how to enter a "social world" such as a hospital, how to make his or her way through it (without creating too much havoc) and how to get close enough to the regular inhabitants to understand how they see their world. At the same time the observer learns how to avoid identifying too much with the observed and with their perspectives. It is no wonder that sociologists talk frequently about "entry" and "departure" from the "field," for the borders between participation and observation are continuously crossed. And though sociologists must come to know the worlds they study in very familiar terms, they have to be constantly mindful that they have come for a while in order to watch, and not to stay. There is a special poignancy to the "hands across the seas" feelings of intimacy and friendship that arise in the course of doing field research, for the time-limited closeness is all the more touching because, for a short while, it brings people together who would ordinarily never come to know each other so well.

For the observer, it is not simply a matter of standing back, uninvolved, for when we join our subjects in their rounds of life we necessarily play at being one of them, and in fact may be mistaken for one of them (in my case, simply by putting on surgical clothing). Furthermore, it is usually easier for everyone concerned if we act like part of the group, although we occasionally offend by making ourselves too much at home or overstaying our welcome.

The reactions of our subjects vary widely: some receive us with cool suspicion and hostility, and others affectionately offer us "insider" roles such as mascot, honorary visitor, or "resident sociologist." Thus, although there are barriers that are never broken, there are strong forces to draw us into the worlds we study. For every world has its own prescriptions for experience, its own interpretive and moral framework. Every social world has its own rules about what is to be attended, and how. To be a participant or insider means that one is guided by this socially shared "definition of reality." Thus, doctors come to see things in ways which are consistent with their particular positions and interests in their world. A surgeon comes to believe in the efficacy of surgery; a medical doctor in the efficacy of medical therapy.

To be an observer means that one is not guided by the same rules of attention and interpretation taken for granted by those on the inside. Thus an observer watching an angry resident who is roused from sleep to examine a sprained ankle in the Emergency Room in the middle of the night need not share the resident's interpretation that the patient is "crazy" or "abusive." I believe that in order to do good sociology one must be willing to make deep excursions into the world under study, yet still remember that one is there not to join it but to watch.

Although most of my time was spent with physicians, and particularly surgeons and surgical residents, I also observed nurses and orderlies in some detail and came to some understanding of their own perspectives. In addition, during a period of several months I separated myself from the staff and instead followed the experiences of patients (primarily those who were undergoing cardiac surgery) and their families. During this portion of the research, I introduced myself to the patients and families as a sociologist who wished to understand the hospital from their point of view, and in many cases I paid daily visits to patients throughout their several-week stay in the hospital.

A few words must be said about how I have disguised the identity of the hospitals and individuals. The hospital named "Lakeside" is actually a composite of three hospitals where I did research. The hospitals were located in different parts of the country and ranged in size from approximately 350 beds to well over 600 beds. They were all private, "non-profit," teaching hospitals associated with prestigious medical schools, and they were all located in metropolitan areas. All the hospitals had a medical staff composed of private attending physicians, house officers, and full-time senior staff members. All had an active cardiac surgery service. Two of the hospitals drew most of their patients from the local metropolitan area, and the largest hospital drew many of its patients from a wider region. Although the three hospitals varied in some matters (for example, in the relative power of their various subgroups) I was most interested in the situations and features common to all. Observing more than one hospital enabled me to distinguish the common features of hospital life from those idiosyncratic to any one institution. My purpose in presenting a composite portrait rather than distinguishing among the three institutions, then, stems partly from my focus on shared characteristics and regular patterns of hospital life, and partly from my wish to provide maximum disguise for the individuals described. All the names and some of the biographical characteristics of the individuals are changed. Any coincidence of names used in this book with those of actual doctors, nurses or patients is completely accidental.

I have purposely avoided using any sociological references or footnotes in the chapters in order to make the book more readable and involving. However, my research and writing have been deeply influenced by the work of others, and other investigators have reported similar findings. I review some of these works in the Conclusion and Suggestions for Reading.

I am grateful to the University of California, Santa Cruz, for allowing me a two-year leave of absence from my teaching job so that I could carry out this research. I am also grateful to the National Endowment for the Humanities for a nine-month Faculty Fellowship for Research in Science, Technology and Human Values (#F-74-257), which supported me during part of my leave time.

There are many friends and cclleagues who have helped me enormously in the course of this work. I would like to give special thanks to Nancy Adler, Arlene Kaplan Daniels, and Philip E. Slater as well as Dane Archer, John Brockman, Samuel Chase, Todd Gitlin, John Kitsuse, Arnold Milstein, Charlotte Green Schwartz, Anselm Strauss, Norma J. Wikler nad Irving K. Zola. I would also like to thank James Landis for his editorial advice and Douglas Pinto for his explanations of technical questions.

Most of all, I am grateful to the many doctors, nurses, and patients who generously allowed me to enter their worlds, even when my presence must have been a painful thorn in their sides. In the case of the medical staff I am especially appreciative, since they must have suspected or even known that I would be taking a critical view of many of their activities. I am particularly sorry that I cannot thank these individuals by name, because they are the ones who have made this research possible. Nonetheless, I hope they will recognize my deep appreciation.

M. M.
February, 1976

PART

I

_____ 7

COMPETITION AND CONFLICT
WITHIN
THE HOSPITAL STAFF

CHAPTER

1

THE ULTIMATE IN SURGERY

MR. BERNSTEIN WAS lying on a stretcher, still awake but heavily tranquilized in preparation for open heart surgery. He had been left alone in a quiet corner of the Operating Room corridor and was already dozing on and off into a deep sleep. In the room where his surgery would take place, two orderlies, one a young man and the other a fiftyish, heavyset woman, were alone and silent, cleaning up the remains of the previous operation and readying the room for the next case.

The anesthesiologist hurried by, made a brief check of his patient, and looked through the windows of the doors into the operating room. He glanced restlessly at the clock on the wall as he watched the woman clumsily stooping at the base of the surgical table, giving it a weary and per- functory dab with her wipecloth. He had complained many times that the housekeeping personnel simply did not under- stand the importance of cleaning the operating rooms. He pushed through the doors and burst into the room. "Come on, come on, let's get the show on the road." With a gracious smile he picked up a mop and vigorously spread it across the floor, pushing especially hard at the large dried-up blood stains on the back tile. The woman stopped wiping and tried to take the mop from the doctor's hands, but he told her to finish what she was doing.

Several young, trim nurses arrived, and they moved hastily and quietly, setting up the equipment that would be used in the case: poles for intravenous bottles, tables covered with neatly arranged surgical instruments, piles of sterilized drapes and towels, electrical equipment to shock and monitor the heart, and the pump-oxygenator through which Mr. Bernstein's blood would be circulated during part of the operation. The room had the aspect of a house being readied for a party in the last few minutes before the guests arrive.

Mr. Bernstein, a forty-five-year-old shopkeeper who had recently suffered a moderately severe heart attack, was wheeled into the room and quickly put under anesthesia. The nurses pulled back the sheets and his body was painted with a yellow antiseptic liquid. Within ten minutes he was connected through several lines and tubes running from his arms, neck, mouth, legs, chest, and penis to various bottles, poles and monitors. At last he disappeared from sight under the green drapes, with only a square foot of chest, covered with sterile plastic, showing through and framed by the hole in the green cover.

Someone switched on the stereo, and the theme song from *A Man and a Woman* drifted across the room, blending with the sounds of several conversations taking place simultaneously in the room. One pair of surgical residents stood at the foot of the table. They were already opening up a thigh to remove a segment of vein that would be used to bypass the occlusions in Mr. Bernstein's coronary arteries. A different pair of residents more advanced in training (by a year) were at the chest: cutting through the flesh, cauterizing the wound, grinding through the sternum with an electric saw, spreading apart the rib cage, cutting through the pericardium (the sac surrounding the heart), and, finally, exposing the beating heart. Soon that beat would be stopped in order to allow for precise cutting and sewing, and Mr. Bernstein's blood would be detoured through clear plastic tubing into the mechanical pump at the foot of the bed, where it would be oxygenated and returned to his body.

At the patient's head, the anesthesiologist and a resident watched the cardiac monitors and talked about the benefits of various new drugs coming out on the market. A couple of salesmen from a surgical supply company had joined the group, dressed like everyone else in green surgical garments, masks, caps, and shoe covers. They had come to demonstrate a new suture gun that could shoot large wire staples for closing up wounds in much less time than it took to sew stitches with needles and thread. They stood in a corner of the room with their arms folded, occasionally joined by a resident, and discussed the surgical equipment being used in the case.

This surgery, the third open heart operation done that day at University Medical Center, was going very smoothly. The residents effortlessly made all of the preparations for inserting the vein grafts around the occluded portions of Mr. Bernstein's coronary arteries. When it was time to sew the grafts into place, they had an orderly page Dr. Mann, the cardiac surgeon who was in charge of the case. He was upstairs making rounds of his other patients in the hospital.

When Dr. Mann entered the room, the volume of the music was turned down and conversations tapered off. Dr. Mann had the reputation of being a "real gentleman" in the operating room: he never raised his voice or screamed at the residents or the nurses. He was a cool, easygoing fellow who liked to keep things relaxed and friendly. Of all the senior cardiac surgeons he was the most popular among the residents. He was an expert skier and generously allowed his favorite residents to use his weekend house in the mountains when he wasn't using it himself. On one occasion he had explained his philosophy about surgery: "I always say, if it's not relaxed and enjoyable in the operating room, then it's not worth doing. The mood in the OR depends on the surgeon. The surgeon sets the tone. You know, surgery can be the most relaxing thing in the world, when things go smoothly."

Dr. Mann quickly and easily placed the tiny stitches around the two bypass grafts. The heart was shocked back into a good beat with the sterile electrical paddles on the first attempt, and Dr. Mann quietly left the room to finish his rounds. Now that the heart was beating again and Dr. Mann had departed, the mood lightened and someone turned up the stereo again, this time slightly louder than before. An orchestral version of "Moon River" filled the room, and the male orderly tried, unsuccessfully, to make a date with one of the nurses. When the anesthesiologists shifted the subject of their conversation from sailboats to shotguns, the orderly joined them. He teased them about their choice of music, asking why they didn't listen to something more sophisticated, like jazz. The resident answered seriously, "Oh, we listen to rock and classical too, but I prefer 'easy listening'; it sets a nice mood in the operating room."

After the residents had wired shut the split halves of the sternum, they invited the salesmen to step up to the patient on the surgical table and demonstrate the suture gun. Each of the residents tried the gun for a few moments, and they joked about who could shoot the straightest staples. When the wound was closed and Mr. Bernstein finally uncovered from under the drapes, the Chief Resident solemnly nodded his head and said "thank you, gentlemen" to the others. Mr. Bernstein was moved back upon a rolling bed and escorted to the Intensive Care Unit, doing nicely, with a crooked line of staples running down his chest.

But across town, at a smaller hospital, another cardiac surgeon was setting a very different tone in the operating room. As one of the anesthesiologists had predicted the day before: "It's going to be like the War of 1812 in there."

When Paul Lever arrived at Lakeside Hospital at 6:12 A.M. it was still dark outside. Being the surgical intern on the thoracic (chest) service, he had to make quick morning rounds of all the patients who were in the hospital for heart or lung surgery. Some were still having diagnostic tests and others were in various stages of recovery from their operations. They were spread out over several different floors in the hospital, so Paul had to run through the halls in order to get to the operating room by seven o'clock, when he would help the anesthesiologist prepare Mrs. Bergen for her surgery. He had looked into the patient's room before she was taken to the OR, but she was practically asleep from preoperative medication, so he hadn't disturbed her.

Earlier in the week Paul had told the resident he worked

with that he felt uneasy about this operation because he knew that Mrs. Bergen was reluctant to have the surgery. The case had been discussed rather heatedly at the weekly cardiac conference, and Paul's surgical supervisor, Dr. Thomas Dalton, had made a strong case for the surgery. Dalton had asked one of the cardiologists (a medical, as distinguished from a surgical, heart specialist) at the meeting to perform a preoperative diagnostic procedure called a catheterization on Mrs. Bergen in preparation for the surgery. But the cardiologist had objected to the idea, arguing that he was not convinced that the possible benefits of the surgery outweighed the risks in the Bergen case. She was in a debilitated state, so chances were seven in ten that Mrs. Bergen would not survive an operation to replace two valves in her heart, and without the surgery she would probably live for six months to a year. Dalton, the surgeon, did not like being challenged, and he complained: "Oh, I know some criticize us because our statistics look bad, but after all, are we here to help the patients or have good statistics? No, I know that we can fix her up and give her ten good years and I think we should."

The cardiologist, however, had continued to object. There was no point in doing the diagnostic procedure, he argued, because the patient didn't want to have surgery. "She's not going to agree to this operation. Her family doctor told her that if she consents to surgery she's signing her own death certificate."

Dr. Dalton appeared to be irritated, but he persisted. "Oh, she'll have the surgery. I very rarely have a patient refuse me surgery." As Dalton drew the meeting to a close he concluded, "No, I want to help this lady. I *want* to do the operation if we can help her, and I believe we can."

Dalton was unaccustomed to resistance. He had made many important contributions to medicine over the years, and he was a prominent cardiac surgeon whose patients traveled long distances to see him. Those who worked closely with him, however, agreed that this aging medical celebrity was past his prime as a surgeon. He received very few referrals for surgery from the other doctors at Lakeside, and relied upon his reputation and the patients he had treated before for his current cases. Many of the younger doctors found it difficult to argue with Dalton. Because of his renowned achievements he commanded a great deal of respect, and even as he aged he had not lost his ability to dominate every situation with his sharp tongue and dramatic style. Most of the doctors at Lakeside admitted that they were afraid of Dalton and his caustic outbursts, and few refused him anything. It was only in the last few years, when his competence was reportedly slipping, that he had encountered any resistance at all.

As for the Bergen case, under Dalton's orders Paul Lever had booked the operating room for the case even before the advisory conference with the cardiologist had been held or before talking to the patient. Getting Mrs. Bergen to sign the consent form was not difficult. When Dalton heard that the patient didn't want to have the surgery but that her family was in favor of the operation, he declared that she was mentally "too obtunded" because of her medical condition to make a proper decision, and he called a family conference in the hospital. Paul had spoken briefly to Mrs. Bergen the night before the family meeting was to be held, and she had asked to know her chances of living through the operation. He had stated the matter as optimistically as he could: "Well, forty people out of a hundred having your operation would make it through." She had started to cry then, and told Paul that since her children were grown up they didn't need her to live beyond the year. But she wasn't ready to die the next day, so she preferred to settle for six more certain months.

As Paul later explained, he felt uncomfortable in these situations. He felt sorry for Mrs. Bergen, but her life could not have been very pleasant as it was. And, since she was Dalton's patient, he felt that he had no right to encourage the patient to resist her doctor's recommendations. Two hours after the family meeting, Paul heard that Dalton had gotten his way: Mrs. Bergen had yielded to family pressure and agreed to the operation.

On the morning of Mrs. Bergen's surgery, Paul finished his rounds quickly, made notes on what had to be done for the patients on the floors and hurried to the operating room, a little late. The operating room is a small world in itself, set off from the rest of the hospital. A sign on the outer door warns: OPERATING ROOM—DO NOT ENTER, and not far inside is a nurses' station where someone is always sitting to make sure that outsiders do not wander in. Just beyond that desk are the lockers and dressing rooms: separate ones for nurses, orderlies and doctors, but female doctors must use the nurse's room because the doctor's room is for men only. In the dressing rooms street clothes are removed and replaced by green surgical clothing and disposable masks, caps and shoe covers. The men wear two-piece pajamalike suits with a drawstring at the waist; the women wear surgical dresses or a tunic and pants suit. Instead of wearing shoe covers, several doctors and nurses keep a special pair of canvas shoes, or clogs, or Dr. Scholl's sandals in their lockers for wear inside the operating room. The clothing is loose and comfortable. Bare arms and legs are exposed in the clothing, and many stand in their clogs or sandals in bare feet.

Once dressed in surgical garments one can proceed further through the suite into the actual operating rooms, which are arranged side by side along the main corridors. Surgeons and scrub nurses (the nurses who hand materials to the surgeons) also stop at a sink in the corridors and scrub their hands and arms for several minutes with a special soap. Immediately after scrubbing, the surgeons are helped into sterile overgowns that snap in the back and into sterile gloves. Thereafter they are "untouchable" and may not come into physical contact with anyone who is unscrubbed for the duration of the surgery. Their hands and torso may come into contact only with the operating field around and including the surgical wound area and with the sterilized instruments, until the surgery is completed.

Anesthesiologists and circulating nurses (nurses who do various odd jobs in the operating room, not directly in contact with the surgical field) generally do not scrub or wear sterile overgowns and gloves. The anesthesiologist will touch only those portions of the patient that fall outside of the sterile draped area (in cardiac surgery, the anesthesiologist touches only the head and neck once the surgery is underway). The anesthesiologists and circulating nurses must be careful not to come into physical contact with the surgeons and scrub nurse.

The operating room is inhabited primarily by four types of personnel: surgeons (and surgical residents and interns); anesthesiologists and nurse anesthetists; OR nurses and technicians; and orderlies. Members of each group tend not to mix very much with members of the other groups because of the pronounced status differences in the surgical hierarchy.

On the morning of Mrs. Bergen's operation, Paul changed into surgical clothes but did not scrub immediately. Instead he offered to help the anesthesiologist prepare the patient for surgery. He was doing this on the instructions of Dr. Dalton, who was annoyed that the anesthesiologists were so slow in setting up the patients. Dalton had requested that the anesthesiologists come into the hospital at six o'clock instead of their customary 7 A.M. when there was an open heart case on the schedule, but the Chief of Anesthesiology had refused to make special arrangements for Dalton's cases.

As Paul helped the anesthesiologist insert the arterial and venous lines for pressure measurement during surgery, he looked up to see Eric Stoller come into the operating room. Eric had been the senior resident on the service for four months, and this was to be his last day in the hospital; on the following day he would be "rotated" to a surgical service in a nearby hospital.

Eric was a sociable fellow: whenever he entered a quiet room he would try to get a conversation going. As usual, he wore his surgical pants a size too tight. Before scrubbing he gave a little slap on the back to Mary, the cardiac surgery scrub nurse.

Mary was a youthful-looking woman of about forty, but

she kept her age a secret despite frequent teasing. She cut off the bottoms of her surgical dresses to make them short, and she would also call attention to her body in the operating room by snapping the back of her bra, or stopping her work (when she was not scrubbed) to scratch or massage her legs. One of the interns from a previous rotation had remarked on the contradictions of her behavior. On the one hand she would make herself vulnerable by flirting with the young interns and residents and by indicating that she was available. But when she was in the presence of the younger OR nurses she would act very tough, and, sitting in the OR coffee lounge she would loudly boast about her drinking, her sex life and complain of her recurrent cystitis. She had been at Lakeside longer than most of the other doctors and nurses and she had become very protective about the operating room. She treated newcomers and visitors—such as nursing students assigned to spend a day observing in the OR—with such hostility that one of the surgeons had described her as "a mare better left alone with her foal."

While Eric and Mary scrubbed the body and arranged the drapes, they teased each other about being glad that this was the last day they would have to work with each other. Paul and the anesthesiologist remained silent until they completed the insertion of the lines, then Paul left the operating room in order to make a final check on the patients in the Intensive Care Unit.

Jerry Mandel was the anesthesiologist assigned to the case, and he was not very happy about it. He hated working with Dalton, as did all of the anesthesiologists, and so they took turns so that no one would have to do it more than once every two weeks. Jerry was about thirty-five years old, and since finishing his residency a few years before, he had spent most of his time working in the operating room of Lakeside Hospital. Although he sometimes had to work at night, his time off was generally uninterrupted. He worked fewer hours than many other physicians, and this was one of the reasons he had chosen the specialty. The work was fairly interesting, and in an ordinary day he was generally assigned to two or three cases, some of which he took care of himself and some of which were really managed by a nurse anesthetist who worked under his supervision. On the days of Dalton's open heart operations, however, the one case was the only job assigned to the anesthesiologist for the entire day. Dalton's operations were usually very long, and the double valve replacements (such as they were doing on Mrs. Bergen) could take him all day.

Lisa, an anesthetist who would be helping Jerry when things got busy, stopped by to console him for having been assigned the case. He looked pleased to have some company, and he agreed that it was a terrible case to have drawn: "Even if the patient lives, it's going to be very rocky and Dalton's sure to carry on all day." The two discussed the big fight that had occurred the previous week between Dalton and one of the other anesthesiologists, Naga Basu. Jerry Mandel speculated that Dalton always gave Naga a particularly hard time because Naga was from India, and Dalton hated foreign doctors. Jerry supposed that working with foreign doctors was very upsetting to Dalton because it reminded him that he had slipped from more powerful days when he worked with only the cream of the American doctors.

An intern who would be joining the surgical service the next day entered the room. Surprisingly self-confident for a new intern, he stepped over to one of the pretty nurses who worked at the pump-oxygenator and introduced himself. Mary noticed their conversation and glared at them. She had frequently expressed her displeasure with the attention that was lavished on the "pump girls." Asserting her authority as the scrub nurse, she walked over to the intern and demanded to know who he was and what he was doing in the room. The intern turned his back to her, ignoring her remark. She flushed with anger and continued: "You see that door over there?" She pointed to the doorway to the corridor. "Will you please step outside, you're in my way." The pump nurse began to protest, but the intern laughed and left the room. As he stepped over the threshold of the doorway he pointed to the floor and looked from Mary to the pump nurse, saying, "It's okay, she just wants to pee on that line to show whose turf this is."

Jerry Mandel, standing by the patient's head, looked up at the clock, since monitoring the passage of time was one of his responsibilities. It was ten o'clock, and Eric and Juan Mendez, the thoracic surgery fellow from Argentina, were just beginning to "cannulate" the patient's heart: they were inserting large plastic tubes into the major blood vessels; these tubes would carry the patient's blood to and from the pump oxygenator at the foot of the table. This was a tricky part of the operation, as far as Jerry was concerned, because if the heart went into an irregular rhythm now, they were still not prepared to transfer the functions of the heart and lungs over to the pump. There was a sudden quiet in the room and Jerry looked up. Dr. Thomas Dalton had arrived.

His appearance was disappointing. He was an ordinary-looking man, on the verge of looking elderly. At first glance, only his erect bearing suggested his extraordinary character. He might have been called barrel-chested; one of the doctors in the hospital had put it less kindly and said he looked like "a stuffed pigeon."

"Well, friends," he greeted everyone in the room, glancing around as if to take stock of who was there, and meeting everyone's eyes momentarily. "How are things looking?"

Juan and Eric nodded their heads and mumbled something incoherent as they continued to work on the cannulae. As Mary helped Dalton into a sterile gown, vest and gloves, he looked over at the chest and remarked, "I see we're still not cannulated by ten-fifteen, as is our custom." Everyone recognized his sarcasm. He had told the residents over and over that he wanted the patients to be cannulated by the time he arrived to work on the valves. Now he would have to stand around and wait until they were ready. Dalton paced up and down the room, behind the residents. "Come on, boys. We should be moving like bats out of hell." He turned to the new assistant scrub nurse: "Well, young man, you're the fellow Mary told me about. Well, have a good look today and I hope you like what you see—it's the ultimate in surgery."

There had been a controversy about hiring this new scrub nurse. Dalton had announced at a cardiac meeting that he wanted Mary to train a whole new "elite guard" of nurses to work on his operations. The department of nursing had told him that he would have to use the same nurses as all the other surgeons, and they would be assigned as they were available from the daily pool. At the meeting he had argued that his surgery was more difficult and complicated than anyone else's and he needed specially trained assistants. He produced considerable laughter at the meeting when he described how, during one operation, he had been forced to scream constantly at an inexperienced technician who had been assigned to help him. The fellow had come to him later with tears in his eyes and said, "Dr. Dalton, I can't stand this anymore." As Dalton told the story, "I looked at that teary-eyed little fellow and I said to him, 'I can't stand it either.' I ate him up like hamburger."

Having made his point, Dalton insisted that sending unspecialized nurses into his operating room was like "throwing sheep to the wolves." The Operating Room Committee had finally yielded and allowed him one new scrub nurse, and the young male nurse had been chosen to work with Mary.

A few minutes after Dalton arrived for the Bergen case he was joined by a Japanese man whose abundant flesh was straining the seams of his surgical suit. "Look up, everybody. But don't move," Dalton announced. "This is Professor· Shumate, who is visiting from Japan. I told Professor Shumate that we would let him look at how we insert our valves." Shumate did not seem to understand English, but he smiled at everyone when his name was mentioned. Dalton steered the huge man over to Jerry Mandel. "Here, Dr. Mandel will let you stand on his platform and look." As he handed Shumate over to Mandel's care, he shook his head and took advantage of the visitor's inability to understand English. "He's a petite little fellow, Dr. Mandel. He won't take up much of your space."

Dalton peered over Juan's shoulder, just as the young man was completing the attachment of the cannulae. "Juan, how many times have I told you that you *must* wash your gloves every hour. Every single hour. I can't seem to get you to understand that concept. Now, tell me, are you really satisfied with those stitches you're making?"

Juan mumbled, "Yes, sir." The dark, quiet fellow struck a respectful look, but he seemed to pay no attention to Dalton's interruptions as he kept working. He had explained to Paul Lever some days before that he had come to the United States to learn cardiac surgery and he had made up his mind to simply ignore the way that Dalton treated him. "Are you *absolutely* sure that you have healthy tissue under those stitches, Juan?" Dalton persisted: "I know you say so, so I suppose I'll just have to take your word for it."

Stepping back from Juan, Dalton looked more cheerful. It was obvious that he believed the best way to get high-quality work out of the residents and fellows was to breathe down their necks. During the last operation Dalton had found fault with the residents almost continuously, and when a nurse had come into the room to tell him that he was wanted outside for an important telephone call, he had turned his eyes upward towards the ceiling and dramatically implored, *"Someone* keep yelling at them."

Juan was still securing the cannulae, so Dalton turned to the intern who was watching the operation from the other side of the room. "How are things going up in the Intensive Care Unit, Paul?"

"Mrs. Rodgers is complaining of pain from her pacing wires, sir."

Dalton shook his head with annoyance. "I don't know what to say about that. Our patients are always bellyaching about those pacing wires. They say it hurts where the wires are left in. I don't know whether it really hurts them or it's just that they know the wires are there."

He questioned the intern again: "Is Blackwell still killing our ICU patients with overtreatment?" Paul smiled and didn't answer. Blackwell was an anesthesiologist who had just been hired to supervise the Intensive Care Unit, where all of Dalton's patients were sent after surgery. Blackwell had been defying, in unprecedented fashion, the orders that Dalton had left for his patients. Most recently, the arguments between Dalton and Blackwell had focused on their disagreement about how much respiratory assistance should be given to the patients postoperatively. Blackwell was in favor of being very aggressive with the treatments and Dalton had objected that he wished Blackwell would leave his patients alone.

Dalton might have noticed that the intern did not share his critical opinion of Blackwell, for he added, "I don't like to twist his nose, boys. But we really must saddle him."

He asked about the other patients who had not yet had surgery. "What about that woman on the eighth floor, boys? Has she had her x-rays yet? Or are the cardiologists holding us back again?"

"No, she hasn't had the x-rays yet, sir," Paul answered.

Dalton replied angrily: "I tell you, they don't have to worry about anything happening to her in surgery. She's going to die of old age up on the eighth floor, waiting to be x-rayed."

He peeked over Juan's shoulder again. "*Someone* doesn't know how to use that clamp. Shame on you, Juan. That's second-year medicine. For Christ's sake, don't be so rough with that, Juan. Can we *please* try not to tear out the AV groove the way we did last week? That was pretty grim last week, I'm sure you'll agree, Juan, and we certainly don't want to repeat *that* performance."

Jerry Mandel took Lisa to the side and whispered about what had happened in the case the week before. It was the case Naga had been assigned to. One of the surgeons had sliced too far while cutting into the patient's valve. The surgical knife had accidentally sliced right through the myocardium (heart muscle) up to the aortic wall of the heart. It took them hours to patch up the huge tear, and after all that trauma to the heart and the destructive time on the pump, they had not been able to get the patient's blood pressure sufficiently elevated.

Things had gone badly between Dalton and Naga right from the start when Dalton ordered the anesthesiologist to take off two units of blood from the patient at the start of the operation. A patient's blood is circulated through the mechanical pump for oxygenation during surgery, but unfortunately the blood platelets become damaged in the process and lose their clotting ability. Therefore Dalton and many other surgeons had found it useful to withdraw some of the patient's blood before surgery and replace it during the operation with bank blood. Then, the patient's blood, having been saved from the destructive trauma of the pump, could be returned to the patient at the end of the operation, when its clotting factor would be badly needed. Dalton had insisted that this reserved blood had to be sent to the refrigerator and cooled during the surgery, or else, he had argued, its quality would deteriorate. Since he characteristically mistrusted everyone else's intelligence and judgment, Dalton was never a man to say anything merely once, and so he had constantly reminded everyone how important it was to keep the blood in the refrigerator. During the operation the week before, he must have asked Naga at least ten times whether he had sent the blood to the cooler.

Naga had been intensely annoyed that Dalton was telling him what to do with the blood, since anesthesiologists believe they know more about blood than do surgeons. So, instead of sending it to the refrigerator that day, Naga had simply stuffed the two plastic bags of blood into the drawer of his desk in the operating room, and he let them sit there during the duration of the lengthy surgery. At the end, when Dalton called for the blood, Naga pulled the packets from out of the drawer. Dalton either saw this, or noticed that the packets weren't cold, for he asked the anesthesiologist, "How long has this blood been in this room?" Naga had looked at him unfalteringly and lied: "a half hour."

Dalton had appeared stunned at the answer but probably was reluctant to acknowledge openly that he knew he had been defied, for he seemed to hedge his rebuke. "We can't have this, sitting here for a half hour. That blood has to be cooled until the last moment."

After the exchange about the blood, Dalton had continued to have difficulty getting the patient's heart to pump efficiently enough to produce a sufficient blood pressure. In response, Naga had suggested that they give the patient a drug called Dopamine in order to raise the pressure. Dalton ridiculed the idea, but Naga persisted, and finally Dalton had reluctantly allowed it, though not without first expressing his contempt for the idea, saying, "Have you ever seen it work? Frankly I don't know whether you're treating yourself or the patient. But if you must have it, go ahead. I don't suppose it will *hurt* the patient."

When the patient's blood pressure began to rise shortly after that, Naga kept boasting and reminding Dalton that it had been the Dopamine that made the difference. Dalton was caustic: "Oh, all right, all right. Everyone has to have their gods, and if you insist on believing in Dopamine, I'm not going to stop you."

The full clash between Dalton and Naga finally broke out over how quickly to let another drug, Protamine, drip into the patient's body. On the one hand, Protamine was badly needed to encourage clotting and stop the patient's bleeding after all the damage and suturing. On the other hand, too rapid a Protamine effect could also cause the dangerously low blood pressure to take a disastrously sharp fall and itself cause bleeding if given too quickly.

Dalton had wanted to push the drug in quickly, nonetheless, because of the patient's dire condition. But Naga had set up a slow drip and paid no attention to Dalton's repeated complaints to increase the flow. Naga was sure he was right about the proper way to use the drug, and he was tired of having a debate each week with Dalton about what he felt should have been a standard, automatic procedure.

Finally, the insurrection had apparently become too much for Dalton to bear, and with one hand he had pushed Naga away from the bottle of Protamine hanging on the pole, and with the other he reached up and opened the clamp so that the Protamine slipped quickly into the patient's body. While Naga watched speechlessly, Dalton had announced: "I don't like running your business for you, but I really can't put up with this." Afterward, Naga had told the Chief of Anesthesiology that he didn't want to do any more cases for Dalton. The chief had reminded him that everyone else felt the same way, so they would all have to take turns putting up with it.

Jerry Mandel was looking at the cardiac monitors when one of the pump nurses suddenly called out, "There's air in the arterial line." Such a situation is very dangerous, for air bubbles escaping into the circulatory system can cause fatal emboli. Dalton became excited. "Well, we have to remedy that fast, fast. Something's wrong and we can't go on like this." The pump nurse called out, "The air is coming up again in the arterial line." Dalton was turning red. "I know I can fix this. I know I can. It must be fixed." Mandel was watching the blood pressure to see whether the air had created any damage yet. He murmured that everything on his end was okay.

Dalton snapped at him. "Will you talk out loud, for Christ's sake. If you have something to say, then say it so everyone can hear. If not, don't say it at all." Mandel's face flushed, and as soon as things quieted down, he stepped out of the room for a few minutes and asked Lisa to take his place. Dalton, noticing Mandel's departure, turned to his surgical team: "I *know* these anesthesiologists want to preside over their work, but in our kind of surgery it is *scandalous* that they don't know what they are doing. They *don't* tell us if they're not doing something we've asked them to do. They order drugs and don't use them. They *should* keep calling out the name and amount of drug they're giving until we acknowledge it, and we should keep calling the name and amount of the drug we want until they acknowledge it. And if that Naga is a Hindu and doesn't want to give drugs, then he shouldn't be doing this kind of work. Did you see how I practically had to force the Protamine out of his hands last week?"

Bill Cameron, the Chief of Anesthesiology, had heard by now that things were heating up in the thoracic room, so he dropped in to relieve the nurse anesthetist. Cameron had come to the hospital a year before, and had turned out to be an assertive and influential member of the staff. Recently, he had begun to make it known that he felt there were serious problems with the cardiac surgery program. Indeed, it was felt by many in the hospital that Lakeside was not doing enough cases to legitimately offer cardiac surgery, and some of the cardiac surgeons were not around the hospital enough to provide adequate leadership and instruction to the residents who were assisting on the cases. When the staff did only a couple of open heart cases a week instead of one a day, it was impossible for the residents and anesthesiologists to gain enough expertise to do a first-rate job.

Although it was not often openly discussed at Lakeside, the rates of success and mortality and complications in heart surgery were considerably better at the major medical centers that did a large volume of these cases. Dalton and some of the others would insist, when the matter was raised, that their high mortality rates meant nothing, for they were taking on riskier cases that other surgeons were afraid to try. Despite these arguments, many of the doctors at Lakeside privately expressed concern that the cardiac surgery mortality rates were higher than they should have been, and for this reason they generally referred their patients who needed cardiac surgery to one of the large medical centers. Many of the doctors believed that the surgical residents were generally very good, and worked hard, but they could hardly be expected to carry off successful cardiac surgery and its post-operative complications with little experience and training.

Still, Lakeside (and some of the other small teaching hospitals in the area) wanted to offer a cardiac surgery program like the big medical centers, because the program brought the hospital prestige. And there was little external regulation to prevent this inefficient and often dangerous (for the patients) duplication of services.

Bill Cameron was not opposed in principle to having a cardiac surgery program at Lakeside, for he certainly enjoyed the challenge and complexity of the cardiac cases. He was merely distressed at the quality of the program, and annoyed by the troubles that some of the cardiac surgeons created for his management of the operating room. Frequently they would schedule an "emergency" case at the last moment, forcing Cameron to push another surgeon off the OR schedule and creating hard feelings all around.

Since there were several individuals in the hospital who were disturbed by the performance of the cardiac surgeons, the hospital had conducted some investigations into the status of open heart surgery at Lakeside. The last committee reviewing the program had reported that the case load was too small to continue effectively as the service was presently organized. In fact, some who knew about the committee's deliberations privately explained that the members were more concerned about the particular surgeons working in the program than they were about the case load. Their reason for talking about case loads was to create some pressure for the resignation of the chief of the thoracic service, without having to criticize him openly or cause him embarrassment. Thus, he could resign for reason of insufficient cases rather than any implied criticism of his work. But so far, this strategy had not worked very well.

Dalton was cordial the moment that Cameron stepped into the operating room. "Hello, Bill. Boys, make some room for Dr. Cameron so he can take a look at what you're doing. Well, Bill, I know you fellows can't see much from there, but everything is going very well. We're a little slow today, but all the world would agree that it's going very well."

Cameron was the only doctor in the hospital that Dalton

seemed to treat with such deference, and some believed it was a pragmatic response to the likelihood that Cameron would be influential in the future plans of the hospital.

Cameron said that he was glad to hear that things were going well. Dalton searched for a topic of mutual grievance. "Bill, do you know about these new requirements for informed consent? Have you read what we will have to go through now every time we want to book surgery? We have to spend twenty minutes, both in our office and at time of admission, having the patient sign away so that he can sue us later. We have to tell them, both in our office and later, how they can have a hemorrhage and a cardiac arrest. This must have been dreamed up by some bureaucrat who has never been in an operating room. It's simply unjustifiable, and everyone knows that no one is fairer than I when it comes to informing about risks."

When Jerry Mandel got back and saw Cameron in his place, he jokingly whispered, "Who let you out of your cage?" The anesthesiologists often teased one another about their subservience to the surgeons. Cameron went off to have some coffee, saying, "I've been fed but not watered."

The second artificial valve was practically inserted in Mrs. Bergen's heart. Installing these valves involved a long and tedious process of placing many stitches around the skirt of the prosthetic device and then pulling on the threads to draw the valve into place. Dalton called to the pump nurse and asked how long they had been on bypass. "Almost three hours, Dr. Dalton." It is not a good thing to keep a patient on the bypass pump for very long, because complications and mortality increase dramatically after the first two hours. Juan and Eric were about to draw the second valve into place and Dalton signaled to the Japanese visitor, who had been watching quietly. "Now I want Professor Shumate to see this valve and how well it is placed." He looked up at the huge, uncomprehending man, and Dalton grinned and added, "You see, nice little Japanese stitches."

He turned to Mandel. "What's the mean blood pressure?" Mandel replied, "Seventy-nine, eighty." Dalton objected: "Oh no, that can't be. Something must be wrong with your measure." Mandel answered, "That's what it is, Dr. Dalton. I've checked it twice."

As Mandel had earlier explained to his assistant, Dalton never wanted to believe that the anesthesiologists were correct when they told him information he didn't like. Mandel had heard that in the hospital Dalton worked at before coming to Lakeside, the anesthesiologists had become so tired of arguing with him about the blood pressure that they installed a special monitor facing the surgeon which they would set permanently at his favorite reading. Meanwhile, they would use an accurate monitor that they kept hidden from his sight. The difficulty now was that Dalton was unaccustomed to hearing figures he didn't like, and when they told him the truth he insisted that they must be wrong. Mandel had come prepared for Dalton today. He had inserted a second, independent device to measure the blood pressure, and the next time Dalton told him that his reading must be wrong, he was going to have the satisfaction of demonstrating the corroborating second measure.

The stitching of the heart had finally been completed and they had begun to redirect the blood flow back into the patient's heart, gradually taking her off the bypass pump. Dalton asked how long they had been on bypass. The pump nurse answered: "It's been three and three-quarter hours, Dr. Dalton."

Dalton appeared nervous about the amount of time that had elasped. "Well, it's been a long run, but it's been a good run. And she has solid valve placement." Since the valve placement was Dalton's special contribution to the operation, he often called attention to the masterful quality of this aspect of the operation.

Suddenly Mandel called out that the blood pressure had dropped from seventy-five to thirty, and he expressed his fear that this was the delayed consequence of the air bubbles that had escaped earlier into the arterial line and that might have finally formed an embolus.

Dalton disagreed. "That blood pressure drop is nothing. Are you sure you're reading it correctly? I don't trust those measures. I'm sure the drop is just coming from warming her up." But Juan and Eric simultaneously noticed that there was suddenly a lot of bleeding around the heart muscle. The heart was bleeding from somewhere. They quickly moved to fibrillate the heart out of its beat again and get the patient back on total bypass so they could find the tear in her heart and repair it. The fibrillator didn't work, and after investigation it turned out to have been unplugged. Dalton's rising voice started to plead: "Come on, folks. It's been *such* a good job. Let's not distintegrate now."

Back on bypass, they had trouble locating the leak because there was so much blood splashing around the heart. Dalton glared at Juan: "I bet someone poked one of his instruments right through her heart." Finally it appeared that a puncture had been made with a surgical instrument while they had been inserting the aortic valve. Dalton was beside himself with anger. "This happens to us too much, Juan. I don't know how to impress this upon you."

Juan had been ignoring Dalton's accusations and appeared to be concentrating on finding the tear so that he could repair it with surgical patches they called "pledgets." Every time Juan prepared a pledget Dalton would find something wrong with the way he was doing it. Finally, Dalton pushed Juan out of the way and started wildly to string up patches himself. While the blood oozed and obscured their view of what was happening, Dalton kept everyone informed. "Well, folks, I don't know if there's only one hole here or more, or where it is. The truth be told, I don't really know what I'm doing. I only hope to God there's a hole where this patch is going."

The repairs would not hold. Once again they had to cut open the heart to locate the puncture site in order to stop the bleeding. Mrs. Bergen had been on bypass for six hours when Dalton felt satisfied that they had stopped the bleeding. He was worried: "Well, folks, I don't know if we're gonna get away with this one, but I hope we do. I *do* want so much to help this woman."

Eric noticed that perspiration was dripping down from Dalton's face, and it was falling dangerously close to the open heart where it could cause contamination. He called to the circulating nurse: "I think Dr. Dalton needs a wipe." She dried Dalton's forehead from behind with a towel, flashing a face for all but Dalton to see that expressed her repugnance for having to do this. Dalton, indicating that he thought it was a silly time to be doing something so frivolous as wipe his face, remarked: "Oh, all right. It won't hurt me and maybe it will make the nurse feel better."

Mandel indicated to his assistant that he had mentally given up on the case a long time before. He was no longer actively watching, but was sitting quietly on his stool behind the patient's head. He was going through the motions of his activities, but he no longer carried any hope for the patient's survival. He knew of no recorded case in surgical history of a patient successfully brought off the pump after as long as six hours, and he saw no chance that it could happen in this case.

They were gradually coming off bypass when they noticed blood slowly and stubbornly oozing across the heart once again. Dalton saw that his meticulous patching had failed. He stepped back from the surgical field, leaned against the wall and crouched down on his legs, holding his head in his hands. He looked up, his face red and sweaty. "Well, friends, I'm almost to the point of despair. We don't have any choice anymore. I think we're just going to have to redo the entire suture line." He stood up and changed into a new sterile overgown and gloves for a final attempt to hold the heart together.

Once the heart begins to shred apart, it is very difficult to keep it repaired. The muscle becomes more and more damaged and increasingly vulnerable to further rips. For the third time, they put Mrs. Bergen back on total bypass, so that they could cut the heart open again and once more repair it from the back. The conversations trailed off. As Dalton began, he thought of the time. "Will someone please phone my wife and tell her to come pick up Professor Shumate. He has no way of getting to our home." In a few minutes the head OR nurse (she was sometimes called the "Chief Bird" and did not have many admirers) stepped into the room to tell Dalton that his wife wasn't home. "Well then, keep calling. The cook will answer, won't she? So tell her to come here and pick him up."

The Chief Bird stood alone in the corner and, appearing to be pleased at Dalton's defeat, smiled a rare smile. Dalton glanced up at her, "And I think someone had better warn that Bergen family that we are in deep trouble."

She watched for a moment longer and then left to find someone to talk with the family. When a patient's survival of cardiac surgery seems doubtful, the family is usually informed of the news in progressive stages, partly to help them adjust to the news and also to avoid an unpleasant scene. First they are told (if possible, by a doctor who knows them) that the patient is doing poorly, but that the surgeon has not given up and is still hard at work in the case. Then, by the time there is no longer any question of the patient's death, the family will already be prepared for the news and less likely to be unmanageable.

The oozing would not stop. Angrily, Dalton pushed Eric and Juan out of the way and stood over the patient by himself. "Okay, now *I'm* gonna do it. I'm certainly tired of everyone else getting in the way. I'm going to sew the rest of this."

Eric and Juan shrank back and silently exchanged blank expressions. Like the anesthesiologist, they expressed through their gestures that there was nothing left to do, but Dalton kept patching. Every few minutes he would look up from his stitching with a hopeful expression and say: "I think we have it now, don't you?" The others, seeming reluctant to argue, would weakly agree.

Finally, Dalton seemed satisfied with the repair and ready to start the heart beating again. He reminded everyone that the heart had responded nicely after the first pump run, before the tear had appeared, and there was no reason why it shouldn't do so again. He called out to anyone in the room, "How long have we been on bypass? Five hours?"

Mandel wearily raised himself from his stool. "No, Dr. Dalton, it's been seven and a half hours."

Dalton made a face of disbelief. The pump nurse repeated the time. "Seven and a half, Dr. Dalton."

He still looked determined. "Seven and a half hours. That means if we get her off the pump alive we will succeed in having the longest pump run yet resuscitated in history. Isn't that right?"

Mandel answered patiently, "Yes, Dr. Dalton. I've never seen it go beyond six hours."

Dalton nodded his head excitedly, up and down. "Well, I think we're gonna make it. She's had good perfusion, hasn't she?" He looked around at everyone in the room. "There's no reason why she shouldn't make it. I think we'll do it. I've closed those holes with good, solid sutures."

At 6:37 P.M. it was at last time to try to shock the heart back into beating, to push it into taking up its work again after all those hours of tearing and cutting and sewing and after being allowed a long period of rest while the mechanical pump had done its job. Eric and Juan grasped the paddles. Everyone stepped back from the table. Dalton orchestrated the application of the current: "One, two, three, *shock!*"

The heart was too tired. There was no response. They increased the voltage of the current and tried again. There was still no response. They turned up the current again, and still there was no response. They tried for a fourth time. No beat was recorded. Finally, Dalton injected a chemical stimulant and massaged the heart with his hands. But the heart would not beat.

Now, there was no longer any delay. Dalton looked carefully around the room at the dozen or so people who had been collected together for the past twelve hours. Without much expression he announced: "Well, I'm ready to quit if you all are." There was no objection. Everyone nodded their heads.

Most had believed the patient was lost hours before, and now they seemed anxious to go home.

Dalton went on: "I just want to say that it's been a tremendous effort you've all shown here today, and you shouldn't feel discouraged."

Mandel humored the surgeon, while everyone else was silent. "Yes, Dr. Dalton, it really looked like we would make it for a while."

Dalton crouched down on his legs again, leaning against the wall, with his face in his hands. He looked up at Eric. "I'm truly sorry that this had to happen to you, Eric. You've been *such* a good resident. You've worked so hard here these four months and I wanted so badly for you to have a good case on your last day."

He stood up, pulled off his gown and gloves, and left the room. Without a word, Juan and Eric started to sew up the chest cavity and Paul and Mary quickly disconnected the lines, tubes and equipment. As they finished their work, Dalton hurried off to his dinner party at home. Those left in the operating room heard him toss his final remark over his shoulder. "It's just not fair. To have gotten so far and done so well, and lose so badly."

2

THE GREAT SAVE

THERE IS A RED TELEPHONE in the Emergency Room of Lakeside Hospital that is used only as a direct line to the city Police and Fire Departments. When the red phone rings, it is a signal that a case of extreme emergency is on the way to the hospital. One Wednesday night at about 10 P.M. the police phoned to say that they were bringing in an unconscious young male who appeared to have taken an overdose of heroin.

One of the Emergency Room nurses had the announcement paged over the hospital loudspeaker that there was a "code" (an attempt at resuscitation) in the ER. Another nurse readied one of the treatment rooms by moving in the code equipment and setting up IV poles. Throughout the wards of the hospital, residents and interns dropped what they were doing and rushed down the stairwells to the ER. As they assembled by the desk they joked with one another about how dull things had been on the floors, and how they had come to take part in whatever little excitement the evening had to offer.

Even before the police car arrived, Dale Richards, the medical resident who was covering the Coronary Care Unit that month, had arrived in the Emergency Room with Daniel Kates, one of the medical interns. It was customary for the resident assigned to the Coronary Care Unit to attend the codes, since many of the patients who survived them were subsequently transferred to the CCU for intensive care. Standing around, waiting for the police to arrive, the resident and intern made bets on whether the case would be a real emergency or just a teen-ager who had swallowed too much aspirin.

But at least, they assured one another, this time they knew it wouldn't be some old alcoholic who would "waste" all of their time in the Coronary Care Unit.

Dale Richards had made it known among the other house officers and some of the staff that he was getting fed up with his rotation at Lakeside. Ordinarily he was a resident at City Hospital, which he enjoyed considerably more, but three times a year he had to do a month-long stint at Lakeside. It was a different job entirely. According to Richards and the other residents, at City Hospital the patients (who were mostly poor and black) were *really* sick and many had unusual or extreme diseases that were interesting for the residents to diagnose and treat. But even more important to the residents, at City Hospital the patients had no private or "attending" doctors to meddle in their hospital care, so the residents like Dale were given a free hand to run the whole show. At Lakeside Hospital, however, Dale Richards complained that the private doctors had ultimate control of the cases, and he felt that the residents were insultingly treated as lackeys who had to do the "scut" work and carry out the orders of the private physicians.

Richards did not accept this reduced status cheerfully. He had openly expressed his opinion that most of the private doctors at Lakeside were either senile, doddering old fools who knew nothing about modern medicine, or else were nervous young specialists in internal medicine, barely out of their own residencies and still getting used to being responsible for private patients. These young ones were the worst, according to Richards, because they treated the residents autocratically in the characteristic fashion of insecure individuals just barely ahead of those whom they direct. But even though the private doctors had the power at Lakeside, Richards had expressed no doubt that he and the other residents were more competent to handle emergencies. Even some of the private doctors agreed that the residents were in their prime years of doing emergency medicine (the residents fondly called it "Guts-Balls Medicine"), for at City Hospital it was quite ordinary to have several cases of drug overdoses to resuscitate each day.

Of all the residents, Richards most often expressed irritation with the private doctors. Earlier in the evening he had one of his frequent arguments with Coleman, an attending cardiologist Richards considered to be one of the most annoying. According to Richards and some of the other residents, every time one of Coleman's patients had a chest pain Coleman would scream that the patient had to be admitted to the Coronary Care Unit for close observation. As the resident covering the unit, Richards was supposed to approve all the admissions (which he tried to keep to an absolute minimum, since each admission meant that he had to personally do a two-hour "work-up" examination). After several run-ins with Coleman about who could be admitted to the unit, Richards had gotten word from the Chief of Medicine that he shouldn't argue with an insistent attending doctor. So Richards had told his friends in the hospital that he wasn't going to bother with anything at Lakeside Hospital: if they didn't treat him with the respect he deserved and loaded him with work that had no teaching value for him, he would do the least work possible. If Coleman wanted to throw his weight around and send all of his patients to the Coronary Care Unit, Richards had complained that *he* wasn't going to "work his ass off for them." He certainly wouldn't do a thorough work-up: instead of two hours, he had threatened he would spend only twenty minutes on each patient.

Several members of the hospital staff had observed Richards' attitude and considered him lazy and arrogant. The image was enhanced by his attractive appearance. Neither his tanned and well-rested face nor his spotless white pants and jacket ever showed the stains and grime of work that were evident in the clothing and appearances of the other residents and interns.

The sounds of the police sirens came closer and finally the police wheeled in a stretcher supporting the well-built but badly bruised and unconscious figure of a young man. As he was shifted from the stretcher to a treatment table, the nurses cut and ripped off all of the clothes from the motionless figure, and the police related what information they had. Apparently he was the boyfriend of a teen-aged girl, now in the Intensive Care Unit upstairs, who had been rushed into Lakeside only the night before, also apparently of a drug overdose.

Dale Richards' friend David Marks, the resident who had resuscitated the girl the night before, was standing by and laughing excitedly, shaking his head back and forth: "This is fantastic," he marveled, "two opportunities to do a Great Save." Like Richards, he had been missing "Guts-Balls Medicine" at Lakeside and was grateful for the long-awaited break in the boring routine of cases involving chronic illness.

Daniel Kates was one of the most aggressive interns in the hospital, and as usual, he had been one of the first to arrive in the Emergency Room after the announcement of the code. He had worked his way into the middle of the action (some of the doctors were doing things to the patient and some just watching). Like the residents, he had often expressed enjoyment at the chance to do a resuscitation, and he had already covered up his clothes with a "johnny" robe and was beginning to do a lumbar puncture procedure in the boy's spinal cord.

As he inserted the needle into the spine he chatted to anyone in the room who would listen. "I missed out on last night's case, but this will make up for it. You know, I've been involved in every single mortality case this year, and this one looks like a good prospect."

Irene, the charge nurse in the Emergency Room, looked annoyed with the intern. "Kates, you are the most morbid person I've ever met." There were others who shared her sentiments. Several members of the staff had privately expressed worry that Kates might be seriously emotionally disturbed, but they didn't know what they could do about it. He was technically a fairly good doctor, but they considered his personality to be distinctly bizarre.

Kates looked up, grinning, his johnny already smeared with blood. "Why do you say that?"

"The way your eyes light up whenever there's trouble."

As Kates proceeded with the lumbar puncture, Dale Richards suggested a different way of doing the procedure. Kates looked annoyed, and even though Richards outranked him by a year, Kates insisted on his way. As they argued about the relative advantages of each method, the Chief of Surgery peeked in through the curtains.

There had been a hospital Executive Committee meeting that night and it was just breaking up. Dr. Douglas, the Chief of Surgery, had walked through the Emergency Room on his way out to the parking lot, and when he saw the crowd around the treatment room he had looked in. When he saw the resident and intern arguing about the lumbar puncture instead of attending to the emergency he appeared to be irritated. He remarked to a surgeon standing nearby that if they had been surgical house officers he would have made a remark, but these house officers were from the department of medicine. Anyway, he conceded to the other surgeon, even though he had an unusually good group of residents during the current rotation, ordinarily the surgical residents were no better than these. As far as he was concerned, most of the house officers behaved like gangs of juvenile delinquents. In order to demonstrate their masculinity they were always daring one another into doing the most drastic procedure available in any situation. Douglas voiced his frequent complaint that residents were not what they used to be when he was young. Nowadays they were slow and lethargic in attending to their work, and they only shifted gears and moved when they saw the chance to do something daring.

But even when he had been a surgical resident, Douglas recalled, there had been pressure to try daring procedures. He had not been popular with the other residents because he was very cautious about taking drastic actions which might be avoided. Even now, as Chief, his conservatism was interpreted by many of the young residents at Lakeside as indicating a fear of doing surgery, and he knew that many joked that he was an anti-surgery surgeon. Over and over again he tried to convince the residents that neither their masculinity nor their surgical competence rested on being quick to do something extreme. At every meeting he would caution them: "You know what they say about the City Hospital resident: he's sure, he's fast, and he's *wrong*." But it was no use, he complained to the other surgeon.

Just the other afternoon Douglas had been walking through the Emergency Room and saw one of the residents performing a fast excision of a cancerous skin polyp from a man's shoulder. As he told the story, he became extremely upset because, for one thing, the resident didn't know what he was doing and he had now increased the likelihood that the malignant cells would spread. But it was also a shock to him that these things were going on in his surgical service. Residents weren't supposed to be able to "book" their own operations in the Emergency Room, and he hated to think of what must be going on in the hospital behind his back.

On other occasions Douglas had also complained that the private surgeons were really no better than the house officers. Many of them, in Douglas's view, were just as stupidly aggressive as the residents (indeed most of the jokes among surgeons were about being made to look like a fool because one didn't take action quickly enough), and half of the private surgeons, Douglas was afraid, were just interested in making a fast buck. As he left the resuscitation team behind him and walked down the corridor of the Emergency Room he met the Chief of Medicine, and the surgeon suggested that the other chief might want to look in on the code.

When Dr. Tanner, the Chief of Medicine, arrived at the code there was a crowd of staff standing in the corridor. Aside from the group of five or six doctors and nurses who were actively involved in the resuscitation, there was an outer circle of kibitzers and the room was filled with interns who were joking about using the code call as a welcome opportunity to get away from the tedium of the wards and the rows of elderly and chronically ill patients who they felt did not deserve to be in the hospital.

Tanner teased one of the interns, "What are you doing

down here, Dr. John? You're always where the action is, aren't you?" His smile showed that Tanner sympathized with the interns and residents. He had often remarked that it was always a disappointment for the house officers to discover that the bulk of medical work involved tedious and repetitious procedures on routine cases.

The patient was still unconscious, and now breathing with the assistance of a respirator pushing air into his lungs through an endotracheal tube inserted into his throat. He had not yet been roused from unconsciousness, and the doctors speculated about the bruises on his head and whether head injury had anything to do with his condition.

There had been some brief trouble getting the endotracheal tube inserted properly. At first, one of the interns had inserted it incorrectly so that air had been forced into the patient's stomach instead of his lungs; they had fortunately discovered their error immediately and corrected it. Such a mistake is not uncommon among inexperienced interns. Some believed that the job should have been left to the anesthesiologists because the only time the medical interns got to practice the procedure was after a patient had just died in the Emergency Room.

Meanwhile, the charge nurse had paged Dr. Lerner, the private attending physician who had taken over the care of the girl friend the night before. The nurse had decided that Lerner might as well handle both cases, and she told the group of doctors that Lerner would be arriving in a few minutes.

Dale Richards made a face of annoyance, and he began to complain to the other house officers. He didn't want any "jerky" private doctor "yapping at his heels" and telling him what to do. He looked up at the Chief of Medicine. "Well, if that private thinks he's gonna run this code while I stand around watching him with my finger up my nose, he's crazy. If he says a word, he can do the whole thing himself."

Tanner laughed sympathetically and said he was going to leave before he got dragged into a fight between Richards and the private doctor. On other occasions he had indicated that he liked his residents more than he did the private doctors, even though he felt that the residents were a bit immature at times. The private doctors were much more troublesome to him than were the residents. Ever since he had become chief of the service ten years before he had run into continued resistance from the private doctors. When he was hired it had been with the explicit understanding that he was to facilitate the conversion of the hospital from a private, community hospital (in which attending doctors had complete autonomy and control) to a teaching hospital affiliated with a nearby medical school (in which the authority was to shift to the residents and interns, the teaching staff, and the program directors). He had been forced to struggle with the private doctors over each bit of change; they had resisted the shift and resented the accompanying encroachments on their power and autonomy. Still, he didn't yet have sufficient power to dictate everything as he pleased, and so he had to keep up good relations with the attending doctors and try to console the residents as best he could.

It was obvious that Dale Richards was burning up at the thought that Lerner would soon be arriving, and Tanner attempted to tease him out of his anger. "Well, Dale, I'll leave it up to you to handle the matter diplomatically. I know I can count on you to be tactful." He laughed and squeezed the resident's arm as he turned to go.

Dr. Lerner arrived just as Richards was pushing the nasogastric (NG) tube down the patient's nose into the stomach. He was dressed in an expensive-looking suit and a brightly colored tie. The residents had often joked that coming to a code wearing expensive clothes provided the private doctors with a convenient excuse for standing back while the residents became covered with blood and vomit. And since (according to the residents) the private doctors knew nothing about emergency medicine, they could stand on the sidelines while the residents did all the work. Then, only after the patient was out of danger, the private doctors would move into position and take little actions to reassert control, such as making minor changes in the orders that the residents wrote in the patient's chart. Still, most of the residents had expressed a preference for the hang-back complaining types over the doctors like Coleman who tried to control every move the resident would make.

Lerner leaned over the resident's shoulder and made a joke about being stuck with two bad cases. He appeared to be nervous and uncomfortable and somewhat uncertain about his participation in the case. Richards looked pleased that Lerner was apparently not going to interfere with the code, and he greeted him warmly, and with amusement requested his assistance. "Dr. Lerner, I'm glad you're here. Could you get some tape for me so we could anchor down this NG tube?"

Lerner fumbled around the supply shelf and handed the resident a piece of tape that was much too short. The nurse moved in and fixed the tube into place.

Richards laughed. "Dr. Lerner, you're an embarrassment to City Hospital, getting the wrong kind of tape." Lerner had done his residency just five years before at the same hospital that Richards worked in most of the time. It was a competitive residency program, well known for turning out excellent doctors, and Richards had often admitted that it bothered him to see how insecure the private doctors became about doing emergency medicine after just five years. It was like looking into his own future, Richards had explained, and it distressed him to think that in a few years a resident would be laughing at *him*.

Kates, the intern, joined in the teasing of Lerner: "Of course he's an embarrassment to City Hospital. He wound up here at Lakeside."

As they tried to assess the seriousness of the boy's condition, the doctors joked about how poorly Lakeside compared to City Hospital: at Lakeside the patients were richer and the setting comparatively luxurious, but it was "Mickey Mouse" medicine compared to what they got at City.

After asking how the girl friend was doing up in the Intensive Care Unit, Richards teasingly asked Lerner if he wanted to take on the second case as well. Lerner made fun of his own nervousness: "What's the blood pressure? I'll only take the case if the blood pressure isn't too low."

Richards seemed cheered by Lerner's willingness to take a subordinate position, and he gallantly told Irene, the nurse, that he would do some of *her* work and insert the Foley catheter into the patient's bladder. As he fumbled with the kit, and had to keep lubricating the patient's penis as he tried unsuccessfully to insert the tube, Richards glanced sympathetically toward the older doctor, looking embarrassed as he surrendered the job to the nurse. He joked to Lerner: "You see how quickly even residents become outdated?"

After further jokes about the competence of each of the doctors in the room, they speculated on the boy's condition. There was a large bump on his face and his left leg showed noticeably less response to stimulation than the right, so they debated about whether there had been any brain injury. By now, the patient, who was very large and muscular, was getting agitated and thrashing about, trying to pull the endotracheal tube from his throat.

The technician from radiology had just arrived and they were about to take x-rays, but since the patient would not lie still, the doctors decided to restrain him first by tying his arms into cuffs at the sides of the table. As Lerner started to tie down one arm, Richards laughingly called out, "Watch out! He's a professional boxer!" Lerner dropped the arm and jumped back, blushing when he saw that the resident had been joking.

Even with his arms tied to the sides of the table, the patient kept jerking up and twisting around, gagging and trying to spit the tube out of his mouth. Irene kept saying that she thought it was because the endotracheal tube simply needed to be suctioned (if too much moisture had collected at the base of the tube, the patient might feel as if he were choking), but no one paid any attention to her.

An anesthesiologist who had joined the hospital staff only days before, specifically to be the new director of the Intensive Care Unit, had been watching from the corner of the room with his arms folded, but now he stepped forward. "Why don't we use ten milligrams of Valium to quiet him so he won't fight the respirator?" No one responded to the suggestion, and the patient persisted in his agitated movements. The anesthesiologist suggested twice more that they use the tranquilizer and finally he directed Irene to administer the drug.

A few moments after the Valium had been given Lerner turned angrily toward the anesthesiologist and argued: "What the hell were you doing giving that Valium without checking it out with me? I happen to be responsible for this patient, you know." The anesthesiologist responded equally hotly that he had warned them three times that he was going to give the drug. Richards stepped back and whispered remarks with Kates. They guessed that this would have to be the new ICU director some of the older surgeons had been describing as an "aggressive young turk."

Prior to this anesthesiologist's arrival, the surgeons had done whatever they pleased with their patients in the ICU, and since few of them knew a great deal about the most current methods in postoperative intensive care, the mortality and morbidity rates in the unit had been quite high. Richards told Kates that he had heard that the Chief of Anesthesiology had purposely found a strong-minded doctor to take charge of the critical cases, so they would not be left to the haphazard postoperative attentions of the surgeons.

After Lerner left the Emergency Room to accompany his new patient up to the Intensive Care Unit, Richards walked over to the new anesthesiologist and introduced himself and shook hands. Having shown some friendliness, Richards then reminded the other doctor that *he*, and not the attending physician, had been running the code. "You know, you really shouldn't have given that Valium when we were still trying to evaluate whether there was brain injury."

Blackwell, the anesthesiologist, looked impatient. "Look, I told you all three times that I was going to do it and no one made any objection until afterwards. If anyone objected, they should have said so before."

Richards agreed. "Yeah, those private doctors are always

hanging back, scratching their heads with their sweaty palms, afraid to do anything until someone else takes charge, and then they criticize you and tell you what you did wrong. They're like little rats in a cage, all frustrated and waiting for you to put your hand in their cage so they can bite."

Upstairs, in the Intensive Care Unit, Lerner was trying to decide whether the boy's brain had indeed been injured by any of the as yet unknown activities that had preceded his arrival in the hospital. He had called Dr. Johnson, one of the staff neurologists, and asked him to come to the ICU to evaluate the situation, and he looked relieved when the other doctor arrived.

Johnson had a hearty manner, and even in the ICU his voice rang out. He stretched his arms around the shoulders of Lerner and Kates and drew them both toward him at the foot of the patient's bed. The patient's left leg had not yet responded much to stimulation. "Let me show you boys some tricks you can use to test if a patient is lying or is really unable to move a limb. You can never trust these addicts, they're always lying so they can get some drugs." Further examination revealed that the patient was coming around some more, and could now move all of his limbs equally well. It appeared that the boy was out of danger.

After completing the examination, Johnson told Lerner that he had a story to tell him, and asked where they could go for a cup of coffee. Lerner looked nervously at the door leading out of the ICU into the hospital corridor. "I don't want to leave the ICU right now. The boy's parents are waiting just outside that door and the moment I step out of the unit they'll grab me and hang on to me."

A nurse standing nearby volunteered: "You can go right in there, in our staff lounge." Johnson eyed the room hesitantly. "Will we be disturbed in there?" "No," the nurse answered, "I'll tell the other nurses not to interrupt you."

Stepping into the lounge and closing the door behind them, Johnson chuckled. "I didn't want to tell you this story in front of the nurses." He poured two cups of coffee, and handed one to Lerner. The story turned out to be a sexual joke that Johnson had heard at a party the night before. As they waited together for another hour to see how the patient was doing, the two physicians commiserated about how difficult it was to collect payments from Medicaid, and how they felt that Blue Cross-Blue Shield payment schedules discriminated against medical doctors in favor of surgeons. In their view, while surgeons were paid large fees by the insurance companies for a suture job that took only ten minutes, as medical doctors they were paid only small fees for diagnosing a problem, such as the one they had that night, which could take several hours of their time. Internists, who generally considered themselves to be the "intellectuals" of medicine, frequently joked that surgeons were the dumb "plumbers" or "technicians" of their trade. But this feeling of superiority did not compensate the internists sufficiently for what they believed to be unfair differences in salaries and earnings. Lerner felt especially irritated about the payment schedules of the insurance companies, for he had many cardiac cases and would often have to spend hours diagnosing and evaluating a heart attack, and a surgeon could earn in twenty minutes the amount of money that Lerner might be paid for a night's work. Lerner and Johnson then discussed the fact that many cardiologists were beginning to administer unnecessary and expensive diagnostic tests because these tests took only a small amount of the doctor's time and brought in a good fee for the doctor from the insurance companies. Many doctors felt that it was one of the few opportunities they had to collect fees approaching those allotted to the surgeons.

About an hour after admitting the patient to the ICU the two doctors left for home, leaving instructions that the patient could be moved out of the Intensive Care Unit the following morning if he continued to improve, which he did.

3

HOUSESTAFF AND PRIVATE DOCTORS: STRUGGLES OVER CONTROL

THE DOCTORS WHO WORK together in Lakeside Hospital fall into three groups: 1) the young "house officers" (interns and residents) who are receiving their clinical training while they provide service to the hospital; 2) the private "attending" doctors who admit their patients to the hospital; and 3) the full-time hospital staff physicians who work on a fixed salary for the hospital either in a training or administrative capacity (for example, as the head of a department or a unit) or in a service capacity to the other doctors (for example, anesthesiologists, radiologists, pathologists). Sometimes doctors in the third group may also have private patients they admit to the hospital, but the bulk of their work involves salaried hospital service.

Between the house officer group and the private doctors there is a fundamental and constantly arising conflict of interests. The two groups do not fight merely out of competitive feelings between generations of doctors. More important, it is the practical interests and realities of their different positions that lead them in opposite and competing directions when it comes to decisions about the diagnosis and treatment of patients in the hospital. Unfortunately, patients often suffer serious injury as a consequence of the conflict between these two groups of doctors.

Pared down to its barest bones, the conflict between the two groups can be described in the following way: it is in the private physician's interest (in matters of finance, personal convenience and legal self-protection) to admit and keep all of his sick patients in the hospital and to administer a cautious and complete battery of diagnostic tests and treatments. On the other hand, the interests of the residents and interns are best served by admitting only a select portion of these patients (those with interesting diseases), by learning and practicing challenging diagnostic procedures on these patients, and by getting them released from the hospital as soon as possible after the diagnosis is made.

While members of each group work daily at patient treatment, they approach their work in the hospital with different aims and interests. The house officers, who work on a fixed salary (usually about twelve to sixteen thousand dollars a year), basically regard their hospital work as the final stage in their medical education. Instead of viewing patients as individuals for whom they are personally responsible, most of the house officers regard patients as cases which may or may not offer an opportunity for learning technical and diagnostic skills, and which demand a greater or lesser amount of unrewarding work. They feel justified in viewing their work this way (as they shall later justify charging high fees) because they have studied and worked for a long time at what they consider to be low wages. While they are interns and residents they prefer to spend their time diagnosing interesting cases rather than attending to routine procedures in ordinary and chronic illnesses. Furthermore, as the number of boring cases admitted to the hospital increases, so does the amount of unrewarding work that the house officers have to do, all on a fixed salary. There is, of course, a minority of house officers who feel personally involved and responsible for what happens to hospital patients, and some even complain about what they regard as insensitive or exploitative treatment of patients by private doctors. However, most house officers, somewhat understandably, tend to think of patients in terms of their teaching value.

Private "attending" doctors who hospitalize their private patients work on a "fee-for-service" basis rather than a fixed salary. They wish to treat their patients as thoroughly and conveniently as possible, and the hospital offers many conveniences: the patients are readily available and waiting in one place; medical insurance companies provide private doctors with a daily visiting fee for each hospitalized case (and these fees can be amassed quickly as the doctor makes speedy daily visiting rounds around the hospital wards); there is a staff of residents and nurses in the hospital who are constantly available to carry out orders and provide twenty-four-hour coverage for the physician; and, finally, the hospital consulting staff provides readily available advice, protection and a diffusion of responsibility should the patient take a turn for the worse. Private doctors are therefore interested in liberal policies with regard to hospital admission and length of stay; house officers are most definitely not.

As the opposing practical interests of house officers and private doctors line up along these basic and conflicting considerations, each group also espouses a set of justifications (which they may sincerely believe) for their own position, while they maintain a more cynical view of the arguments of the other group.

Private doctors argue that *they* genuinely care for the feelings and best interests of their patients, whether or not their cases are interesting; that *they* relate to the patients as human beings and not cases (unlike the house officers); and that *they* want to provide the most thorough and comprehensive care for all their patients. In contrast the house officers complain that the private doctors exploit them as low-paid servants to staff a lucrative hotel-resort for patients who don't even need to be in the hospital.

Somewhere in between these two groups of doctors falls the third group: the physician specialists who work on a salary for the hospital in a teaching, advisory, supervisory or service position. Since these doctors do not generally have many or any private patients of their own, they do not share many of the interests of the private doctors. Instead, they prefer, like the house officers, to centralize authority in the hands of the full-time hospital staff. Furthermore, since they are not heavily involved in clinical practice with private patients, they frequently share the research interests of the house officers. On the other hand, they do share with the private doctors a longer experience, possibly involving a private practice, and a higher status within the hospital hierarchy. They also have long-standing relationships and associations with the private doctors, for they have worked and will continue to work with the private doctors over many years, and with the house officers for only one or two. Thus this third group of doctors sometimes allies itself alternately with one or another of the other two groups, depending on the issue, and sometimes constitutes a separate interest group in its own right.

The conflicting interests of these three groups cannot be fully understood without some historical perspective describing changes in their respective positions over the years in teaching hospitals such as Lakeside.

Before the current shift toward medical specialization, third-party insurance payment plans, and highly technical diagnostic and treatment procedures (all of which require or favor hospitalization of the patient, the use of hospital equipment, and the participation of specialized consultants and technicians), the private physicians who specialize in general or family practice or internal medicine enjoyed unmitigated control over their cases and their practices. They could do whatever they pleased with their patients without having to rely on the cooperation and participation of other physicians or the hospital. In recent times, however, medical practice, technology and organization have changed in such ways that other parties increasingly intrude on the formerly private relationship between the physician and the patient, and the doctor in private practice has increasingly become alarmed about a loss of control, autonomy and money.

This development in medical practice was clearly reflected in the changing organization of Lakeside Hospital. Lakeside began seventy-five years ago as a private community hospital —a place for doctors to install their sick patients who needed nursing care. Gradually the hospital was converted from a private community hospital to a teaching hospital that was affiliated with nearby medical schools and surgical residency programs. Residents and teaching staff were added in increasing numbers every year. The teaching staff and residents were given increasing control by new department chiefs who were recruited specifically to transform the hospital into an institution for research and medical education as well as for patient care. Although private doctors were still nominally allowed control of their cases (to the annoyance of residents and interns), they felt increasing encroachment on their autonomy and territory. The pinch was felt by the private doctors in every direction.

For example, previously, the younger private surgeons and specialists in internal medicine took turns "covering" the Emergency Room, and patients who came through the ER doors without a private doctor were automatically referred to these "covering" physicians. Since the Emergency Room admissions made up approximately forty percent of the total hospital admissions, these cases provided a large share of the business, and gaining referrals in this way was an excellent way for the younger doctors to build up a regular clientele and for the younger surgeons, who had not yet built up an adequate reputation for referrals, to make a lot of money quickly. On an average day in the Emergency Room, a young surgeon could earn several hundred dollars sewing lacerations and examining sprains. A new hospital policy at Lakeside had recently changed this arrangement: patients coming to the Emergency Room without private doctors were no longer likely to be referred to one. Instead, they were seen by house officers under the supervision of the teaching staff (even if admitted to the hospital). These patients and their payments now belonged to the medical or surgical services of the hospital, rather than to the private physicians.

Changes that were inconvenient for the private physicians came with other new policies. Whereas in past years a surgeon could book his operations whenever he pleased and without interference, simply by calling the nursing supervisor of the operating room, surgeons were now informed that they would have to book all of their operations through the office of a powerful staff physician, the Chief of Anesthesiology. This meant that a hospital staff physician was keeping track of their working arrangements, and although he rarely exercised this power, he had the authority to refuse their requests for an operating room. Doctors now found that various committees were looking into their work and reviewing their charts to see whether they ordered expensive tests that were unnecessary, or kept patients in the hospital too long. The committees probably served symbolic rather than practical purposes: few physicians were actually criticized by these review committees, but the idea that a chart might be pulled at random for review, or that a physician had to get special permission to keep a patient in the hospital for more than two weeks, or that the use of many drugs (especially antibiotics, believed to be used too freely by surgeons) required permission from a drug committee, all constituted new invasions into the privacy and autonomy of the doctor.

If these changes were not bad enough, from the point of view of the private physicians, they were merely the beginnings of more to come. Many of the private physicians feared that with the growth of medical centralization and prepaid health plans, they would be squeezed out (financially and in terms of control) even further. Many of the doctors who used Lakeside Hospital had, in fact, recently moved their patients and practices over from another community hospital they had used for many years when that hospital was even more dramatically transformed into a teaching hospital with little power and few privileges for the private doctors. They feared it was just a matter of time before Lakeside would squeeze them out completely (in terms of financial rewards and autonomy). The changes in policy at Lakeside, therefore, caused considerable alarm among the private doctors, for they reflected national trends that were acutely upsetting for physicians in private practice. While some of the doctors were concerned about how these trends would affect their relationships with patients, others were concerned about the monetary implications. Most of the doctors admitted to being upset on both accounts.

Dr. Franklin was a private doctor at Lakeside who seemed less concerned about the financial disadvantages of the new trend than with how the new policies would alter his relationships with patients. Indeed, he displayed such an unusual concern for his patients and lack of worry about money that the other private doctors (who might have pointed to him as a good example of how the private physicians were more concerned with patient welfare than were the full-time hospital staff members) dismissed his behavior with the explanation that he was independently wealthy from a family fortune and could afford (unlike the rest of them) to think about his patients without worrying about the financial aspects of his work. Still, even if Franklin was unusually altruistic, it is important to understand his sentiments, since they were expressed by many of his other physician-colleagues.

Dr. Franklin had recently given up admitting his patients to a neighboring hospital (Town Hospital) and had shifted most of his practice over to Lakeside. He described the reasons for his move in the following way:

"Town Hospital used to be a private community hospital that also served teaching purposes, like Lakeside, but nine years ago it was affiliated more directly with a medical school and a prepaid health plan, and gradually the house officers were given more and more control. The new chief of medicine shifted control to the residents and interns because he wanted to look sympathetic to them so they would be attracted to his residency program, and so he could successfully compete with some of the other teaching hospitals around here for the best residents.

"I've had lots of differences of opinion with the interns there about medical practice. I hospitalize patients for *their* convenience, not the convenience of the hospital staff. One of the fights I had at Town was over the hospitalization of one of my patients who the interns felt didn't 'deserve' hospitalization. She's an elderly woman who lives alone and she had pneumonia and there was no one at home who could take care of her, so I put her in the hospital. The interns got together and held a kangeroo court with a verdict to censure me for my medical judgment in hospitalizing her.

"There was another incident. I had been treating a man for ten years who was morbidly obsessed with his heart disease, which was, in fact, quite minor and insignificant. One day he came to the Emergency Room worrying about his heart, and I examined him there, and I decided that given his psychiatric history, which I had discussed with his psychotherapist, it would be unwise to hospitalize him for heart disease and add to his obsessions. So I suggested that he be treated at home. The house officers, however, who have the final say about admissions at Town, hospitalized him despite my advice and he became so disturbed that he wound up having to be transferred to a state mental hospital.

"Town Hospital is now connected with a community pre-paid health plan and health maintenance organization, and according to their budget, they have calculated that they can't afford to spend more than ten minutes assessing each patient's socio-emotional context. It is also becoming a research-oriented hospital, and this will compromise medical care because you can't drop an experiment in the middle to go see a sick patient.

"Many of my colleagues have also stopped admitting patients to Town in the last two years. One of them recently left after he had a big fight with the interns. He had hospitalized a woman he had been treating for many years. After her admission she had a cardiac arrest and a code was called on her in the middle of the night. The intern refused to call her doctor to tell him about the situation, even after a nursing supervisor insisted that he do it. The patient died early the next morning, and her physician was not informed of her death. To his embarrassment, he learned about it only when he ran into the family the next day in the hospital corridor, as they were arranging for the transfer of the body."

Dr. Sandler, another private physician at Lakeside, more

often voiced some of the other concerns shared by his associates. While he argued, like Dr. Franklin, that patients would suffer if the rights of private doctors were abridged, his remarks also displayed his sensitivity to the financial issues:

"*We* are the patient's advocates, not the residents. They're punitive to the patients who aren't very sick. We want them to get the best treatment, whether or not they're very ill. The residents want to guard the gates in the Emergency Room and not let anyone with chest pain be admitted if they can find a reason not to. If they admit someone through the ER they know that it's their friend [another resident] upstairs who will have to do the work-up, so they're going to look for any reason they can find not to admit the patient.

"And the residents are more interested in getting experience than in caring for a patient. Last week at Mortality Review we talked about a woman who died while taking a stress test for evaluation of her cardiac function. What I wanted to know was, when they tried to resuscitate her, why didn't they give her a ventilating mask right off instead of fooling around with the endotracheal tube? Did she die because the resident wanted to practice inserting an endotracheal tube instead of just giving her oxygen?

"And these prepaid health plans are no good, either. A patient needs to have his own private doctor to watch out for him. Let me give you an example. There's a program going on in the city aimed at detecting hypertension, and lots of people have been screened. One of my patients with high blood pressure was tested and asked to come in, and she was given a prescription to take, and they didn't even bother to check it out with me, even though I'm her private doctor. And it turns out that this patient shouldn't have had that particular prescription because of other health reasons. So I called them up to complain that they should have checked with the private doctor before giving a prescription. And do you know what the project director said to me? He said, 'Don't worry, we're not stealing your patient. We won't take the bread out of your mouth.'

"The doctors in the 'in group' at Lakeside [the staff doctors] who have salaried positions in the hospital are always intimating that all we care about is money, while they're on a low, fixed salary. But they get a free office, and free secretaries. Do you know how much this office costs me? And I have to hire *two* secretaries to try to collect my payments from Blue Cross or Medicare, which I don't collect half the time, or which come in several months late. So when you subtract those expenses from my earnings, I'm earning less than the members of the 'in group' are."

Some of the salaried doctors at Lakeside, however, expressed doubt about Dr. Sandler's claim that money was not the issue in his defense of the private doctor's rights in the hospital. There had recently been some reorganization in the structure of the Psychiatry Unit at Lakeside, and there had been some disagreement about what policy to institute regarding who should be listed on the patients' records as the "doctor" on the case. Since the insurance companies and Medicare would pay for the daily visits of only one attending doctor, the decision would determine who would get the money. Since the Psychiatry Unit was to be governed on the principle of "milieu therapy," the directors of the unit wanted to have the unit or a staff member listed as the "doctor" so that all the money collected from the insurance policies for daily care would then revert to the unit to pay for staff salaries. But several of the Lakeside doctors, led by Dr. Sandler, had objected that it was the policy everywhere else in the hospital for each patient to have a private medical doctor listed on the record as the official doctor, and that such an arrangement was necessary to insure good patient care, even when the patient was admitted for psychiatric rather than medical treatment.

The chief of the psychiatric unit had thanked Dr. Sandler for his concern and told him that even though the "unit" or its staff members would be listed as the doctor on record, he would be delighted if Dr. Sandler and the others would be interested enough to make daily visits to patients in the unit: they were welcome to come as often as they liked.

Sandler had angrily replied: "Well, who's going to pay for it? We won't get paid for our visits and who has the time to come for free?"

Dr. Sandler, if not always completely candid about his financial concerns, was more or less accurate in his analysis of the situation. Most individuals in an ambiguous situation, residents and private doctors included, will defend the policies that maximize their personal interests and minimize their work. It is on the basis of these personal interests that most individuals choose positions in an ideological conflict. The justifications for the position may invoke altruistic arguments (such as sincerely felt claims about what best protects patient welfare) but these justifications are secondary, and most individuals choose positions on the basis of material interests, not abstract ideas.

If one listens to the residents and interns, of course, one hears stories and arguments quite different from those offered by private attending physicians. While many of the private physicians at Lakeside accused the house staff of being selfishly interested only in their own education, and not in patient welfare, the house officers argued that they performed the "slave labor" in the hospital; that half of the time in their hospital jobs was supposed to be devoted to their education, and it wasn't; and that they were not granted the authority, autonomy and respect from the older doctors which they deserved.

Many of the private physicians had argued all along that patient welfare would best be protected not by national, socialized or prepaid health plans, but rather by the traditional private, doctor-patient fee-for-service plan (which now seemed seriously threatened). In recent years, however, some had changed their position on National Health Insurance (just as they had come to support Medicare and Medicaid) when they recognized the profits which could be gained from having the government provide fees for patients who would otherwise have been unable to see a private doctor. Still, they objected to the encroachments on the private doctors' autonomy which some of these programs threatened to introduce. The house officers generally argued that many patients were overtreated by malpractice-conscious or greedy physicians who ordered more tests and procedures than were really needed. Still, the house officers, like the older doctors, did not by and large favor all the aspects of a socialized health plan since they looked forward to the time in the near future when they too would begin to earn the money and independence they felt they deserved after their long years of study.

Finally, whereas the private physicians felt that every patient (provided the bills could be paid) should get the maximum amount of health care, including liberal requirements for hospitalization and the benefit of every diagnostic test and treatment that was relevant, the residents and interns felt that certain categories of patients did not deserve hospitalization and "scarce" medical resources. According to the house officers, the nondeserving included elderly persons with chronic illness who would never get better, alcoholics and other types of patients who were seen as personally responsible for their illness and also unlikely to make good use of medical care, and "crocks": patients who complained of pain or vague symptoms in various parts of their bodies and thus required long and thorough work-up examinations that didn't turn up any medically discernible disorders. Thus "crocks" (also called "turkeys") were viewed by the house officers as not "really" sick and, like the other nondeserving patients, impossible to cure.

The private physicians answered these arguments by pointing out that what the residents were really concerned about was not the rational allocation of medical resources but rather not having to spend their time on undesirable patients who would yield little in the way of esoteric medical education. As the private physicians pointed out, the residents thought it was entirely appropriate to do a "million-dollar work-up" and spend vast amounts of time and scarce resources on a patient with a rare, fatal but interesting disease: a patient no more curable than the alcoholic or elderly, and whose disease, moreover, was so rare that residents were unlikely to gain any skills they would ever use again.

Many of the medical residents and some of the interns at Lakeside felt insulted and demeaned by their subordinate positions, relative to the private doctors. This was especially true of the medical residents who were doing short "rotations" at Lakeside, and who usually enjoyed more freedom and authority at City Hospital. The medical residents were consequently very touchy about (and always on the alert for) any incident that in any way alluded to their lower status. When a private doctor would treat a resident as a less-than-equal colleague, the resident might be angry about it for a long time and complain to the other residents so that the offending doctor would be put on their unofficial blacklist. In some cases, the medical residents even complained about these incidents to sympathetic department heads.

On the other hand, the surgical residents and interns seemed less outraged and surprised by curt orders from the attending surgeons, and more accepting of their subordinate positions. It was their assumption that oppressive and authoritarian behavior from their superiors was unfortunately to be expected and suffered: a staff surgeon who treated them kindly was an unexpected treat to be grateful for. While they might joke and clown around about their servile positions when they were alone, they would never have thought to complain to the Chief of Surgery, except under the most extraordinary conditions.

Unlike the medical residents, who would openly compete with the private physicians to assert superior medical knowledge, the surgical residents were observed to regularly feed information to some of the senior surgeons, all the while making it appear that it was the senior doctors who were the knowledgeable ones. Still, this was a way to demonstrate superiority, for such manipulations could be boasted about with other residents. One resident described the sorts of things he had to do to "handle" a surgeon whom he considered to be brilliant but outdated:

"When I have to call him up at night to report a change in a patient's condition, first I review all the literature on the subject I can quickly get my hands on, and then I repeat this information to him, so he will have all the new research findings at his fingertips and won't have to be embarrassed about not knowing them. Actually, he is often very helpful to me then, because given that information, he can reason much further with it than I am able to, and he can tell me what to do.

"But there are other times when his huge ego creates problems, and he has to be handled very carefully. Last week a patient who had recently had a valve replacement came into the Emergency Room complaining of a severe headache. Dalton thought that she just had an embolus from insufficient anticoagulation for her prosthetic valve, and he said that it was not serious. I thought that she might be bleeding somewhere in the head and in need of immediate treatment, so I mentioned some neurological studies to him that I was sure he wouldn't know, and said, 'I wonder if we should call in a neurologist?'

"He said, 'Neurologists never do any good, so let's not bother.' I think that he had already told the family that it was a harmless embolus, and he didn't want to change the story and let them know that he wasn't sure. At the cardiac conference later that day the situation was mentioned in passing and someone picked up on it and asked what the patient's neurological deficit was. I put it tactfully. I said that I had *just* come from examining her and that the deficit was bigger than the very small deficit that Dalton had seen earlier. This implied that there was bleeding in the head which wouldn't have been obvious earlier when Dalton saw her. Then Dr. Meder said, 'Maybe it's a bleed, and a neurologist should be called in.' So that's how you have to handle Dalton. If you suggest something to him, he'll say no at first, but later he'll say, 'You know, it's funny you mentioned that, because I wrote a paper on that subject in 1942.' Or else later he'll suggest it himself, as if you hadn't. You have to let him think that he's in control, and then he is much easier to work with."

The possibility that the surgical residents were more accepting of status differences was also indicated by the fact that even within their own group they would treat differences of rank very seriously. Whereas most of the medical residents acted as equal fellow-sufferers, in the surgery department the chief resident would literally give orders to the senior resident, and he and the junior resident would issue orders to the surgical intern. As one surgeon pointed out, there is a widely used expression in his field: "In surgery the shit rolls downhill." A cardiac surgeon explained that the different ranks of the house officers in surgery had to be recognized carefully: "When I have to give an order or request information about a patient from the thoracic house officers, I always page them on the loudspeaker using the name of the senior resident. In fact, I *know* it will be the intern who will run the errand of answering the telephone page for the resident, so you might think that I would just page them using the intern's name. But that is not done in surgery. If I don't page the resident's name, even though it is the intern who answers, the resident would be very offended. He enjoys the recognition, and likes being able to send the intern to answer his call."

In thinking about the differences between the medical and surgical house officers, it might be argued that it was the unusual power of the private medical doctors at Lakeside (compared to other hospitals in which they worked) that made their subordinate status such a bitter pill for the medical residents to swallow. But the surgical residents "rotated" through other hospitals as well, hospitals where they too enjoyed more autonomy and authority. It is hard to say why they were less resentful of their reduced status at Lakeside than the medical residents. Possibly, there is a stronger observance of rank and status differences in the general tradition and orientation of surgery than in medicine, or perhaps the circumstances at Lakeside were unique.

Both groups of house officers met with remarks insulting to their status from patients as well as from senior doctors, but again, the surgical residents seemed less offended. When a patient refused to allow the senior resident in surgery to remove her stitches (a task that was considered menial even for the surgical intern four years his junior), and insisted instead that her "real doctor" do the job, the senior resident merely smiled and politely answered that he would inform her private doctor of the request. Another surgical resident, called "boy" by some of the patients because he was foreign, laughed off the insult.

But when a patient began to complain to a medical resident that the hospital food was not being served hot enough, the resident interrupted her and snapped, "I'm not the maître d'." And when, late one night, a patient refused to allow a medical intern to do a simple procedure and asked that he call up her private doctor to check it out first, the intern threatened: "All right, you can ask me to get his approval each time I have to do something for you, but one day when you're dying and needing immediate treatment I'll be on the telephone trying to reach your doctor."

When the medical house officers were particularly frustrated or resentful of the private doctors, they would often take their anger out on the patients. In their daily "Residents' Reports" with the Chief of Medicine, they were implicitly given permission to express complaints about private doctors and patients. In turn, the chief would routinely express sympathy and appreciation for their difficulties, but plead his inability to do anything about changing the arrangements. Almost like the coach of an athletic team, he would boost the morale of his boys, only to send them out into the field for more punishment.

Apart from their function as a complaint station about bad patients and bad private doctors, the official purpose of the chief's daily Residents' Reports was to keep an informal check on everything going on in the medical service of the hospital. Each day the residents would describe the new admissions, and the group would briefly discuss the problematic or interesting cases: most often difficulties in diagnosis or treatment.

Although these meetings were dominated by an outward

show of fraternal camaraderie (both in discussing serious matters and in joking around), the situation was complicated by the fact that although the residents were usually long-term friends and fellow-sufferers, they were also competing with one another for the favor of the chief. For, however much he acted like one of the group, the residents knew that the chief was observing and evaluating them during these meetings, and that his observations eventually wound up in their files and would play a role in what jobs or positions they would next get. Thus the meetings were complicated affairs —on the one hand, competitive and taxing, yet also educational and frequently enjoyable, the latter especially when they were used as occasions to vent hostility against the private doctors and the undeserving patients.

On Mondays, the residents' meetings with the chief were likely to be filled with even more complaints than usual because the natural barriers that guarded admission to the hospital during the week were always lowered over the weekends. As the Chief Resident complained, unnecessary admissions were likely to increase over the weekend because many of the private physicians were out of town on those days, vacationing, and when they heard about a patient who was feeling ill, they would "phone in" the admission for the patient in order to protect themselves lest the patient have an illness that merited hospitalization. Since they were not available to check the situation out themselves, they phoned in admissions for all suspicious cases. Furthermore, over the weekends the surgical admissions were down, since elective (nonemergency) surgery was scheduled only on weekdays. This left several empty beds in the hospital over the weekends, which the administrators were anxious to keep filled for financial reasons, and so everybody (the administration and the private doctors) but the house officers, who had to do the work, had an interest in relaxing the criteria for admissions over the weekends.

On one Monday morning the Residents' Reports meeting was opened by some jokes and complaints about the interns whom the residents supervised. Convinced that they had been much more useful when *they* were interns, the residents complained that the interns covering the Emergency Room had driven them crazy all weekend by repeatedly paging them to come to the ER for advice and consultation. Said one resident: "Every time I turned around to take a piss, I was being paged down in the ER by the intern."

This was followed by some joking about an older attending physician (in his eighties) who had admitted, as was his custom, a patient in her nineties with a chronic disease. She was sure to linger on for weeks in the hospital, requiring countless cut-downs by the residents for insertion of intravenous lines into her collapsed veins, before she would finally die. They laughed about how this doctor would always phone in weekend diagnoses over the telephone (as the chief observed, he seemed to come out of hibernation only on Saturdays), which always turned out to be wrong, and he didn't even bother to come to the hospital, but left all the work to the residents. One resident joked about how the old doctor didn't even know how to read EKG tapes, since his medical training had predated modern medicine: "Once I was in the ER and I asked him if he'd like to look at the EKG of one of his patients, and he snapped, 'I don't read those anymore, Doctor!'"

Next, they complained about a physician who had admitted an overweight forty-four-year-old "girl" who had a hairy face, since the physician felt she might be suffering from Cushing's Syndrome. The chief had been asked to consult on the case, but reporting back to the residents, he laughed, "Oh, she doesn't have Cushing's Syndrome. She's just a fat girl with some bristles. We admit those patients just to see if the Utilization Review Committee is doing its job." The chief had many times indicated that he considered the committee an annoyance and a waste of time.

The reference to Cushing's Syndrome led to a long discussion about one of their favorite topics: the ridiculousness of patients who were overweight. Obese patients were held in contempt by the residents and many of the other doctors, for, like alcoholics, they were viewed as suffering from no legitimate illness but rather were seen to have brought about their own sickness through a lack of self-control, which was considered both humorous and disgusting.

One of the residents asked the others if they knew about Dercum's disease. They did not. "This disease, gentlemen, is a disorder consisting of painful fatty deposits in the thighs of elderly obese women." There were peals of laughter. The resident added that one of his patients on the fifth floor seemed to be suffering from the disease and another questioned whether she also had "bristle" on her face, and might need to undergo tests for Cushing's Syndrome as well.

Next there was more joking about how the patients lied about how much they drank. One resident volunteered: "When a patient tells me that he has just two cocktails before dinner, I know right off that it's more like five." One of the residents described his prize case for the week: a patient who suffered from "Pickwick's Syndrome": a difficulty in staying awake because of extreme obesity creating an insufficient intake of oxygen. There were jokes about using this disease as an excuse to escape from the responsibilities of life, and to escape one's wife, and one of the residents complained, "I'd like to be able to go to sleep myself." When the round-up of new patients was completed the chief agreed that some of the older patients should not be allowed to linger on in the hospital, but rather be transferred to nursing homes. "Let's clean house, boys. There must be plenty of dead wood up there."

Next the residents complained of the troubles they were having with the private doctors who interfered too much with their work. They particularly disliked one of the cardiologists who never let them perform any procedures (such as inserting atrial wires into the heart) on his patients. And if they made a fuss in disagreeing with his opinion, he would always call in the same consultant to settle the matter: a doctor who was one of his best friends. Without fail, the consultant would side with his friend against the resident's position. Since the private doctors, and not the residents, were the ones who could authorize consultation at Lakeside, the consultants were usually used in support of the private doctors' positions.

(Consultants were, of course, also used for their official purpose: to provide another expert opinion in an ambiguous situation. However, still another use of consultation was to provide legal protection for the attending doctor. One internist, for example, was afraid to discharge a patient for fear that a temporary hormonal disturbance might cause her to commit suicide, for which he could be held responsible. He therefore requested a consultation from one of the senior psychiatrists in order to cover himself. The psychiatrist, being very busy, instead sent one of his residents to see the patient. The resident wrote in the chart that he saw no reason to keep the patient hospitalized. Afterward the internist complained to the senior psychiatrist that he was angry about the substitution, since the resident's opinion would do him no good should the patient harm herself. Angry that the senior psychiatrist had not done the consultation, he remarked, "If she kills herself now it will be my ass on the stump.")

The final issue discussed at Residents' Reports had to do with the Psychiatry Unit. The psychiatrists wanted to make the medical residents do the medical work-ups on their patients (since they couldn't and wouldn't do physical examinations themselves) and the residents felt it unfair that they should be stuck with an extra load of worthless (from the point of view of medical interest) cases.

One of the residents explained that he was particularly annoyed because when they had "crazy" patients in the Emergency Room complaining of illnesses they didn't have, the psychiatrists refused to come to the ER to handle *those* examinations. Over the past weekend they had been visited by one of their regular repeaters in the ER who always was sure that he was dying from an asthma attack. They had tried to get one of the psychiatrists into the hospital to see the patient, but the psychiatrist covering that weekend had refused, claiming: "He's just coming in to manipulate me into putting him into the Psychiatry Unit so he can yell at me and tell me how bad I am." This story caused amusement among the other residents. One laughed, "Now, I ask you, *who*'s getting paranoid and defensive?"

As the meeting came to a close they joked about the incompetence of the local Medical Examiner who was too old to bother to do his job. As one of the residents explained, on the rare occasions that the Medical Examiner dropped into the hospital to attend to his business, he annoyed everyone by showing them a set of snapshots of car accident victims that he always carried in his pocket. The residents next told stories about how medical examiners were always lazy and incompetent, and how they were especially likely to allow family murders to pass as natural deaths or accidents. This led to more joking about the shocking things that happen in hospitals. The chief described how when he had been at City Hospital he had discovered a woman trying to suffocate her husband (who was a patient) with a pillow. He had interrupted the incident, and warned the other house officers to look out for the wife, but apparently the next day she walked into the room, drew the curtains around the bed, and finished the job. This story brought to a close the reports for that day, and the residents left the conference room and lingered in the corridor exchanging stories for a while longer before returning to their work on the floors.

If the Chief of Medicine hoped that he might handle the problems of resentment between the groups of doctors in his daily resident's reports, he was not completely successful. Most often these conflicts would indirectly get expressed in terms of the care of a patient, sometimes to the patient's serious injury. As the following case illustrates, when residents and interns are angry with a private doctor, they will often vent their frustration on the patient, for lack of other opportunities to express their feelings.

An intern and a medical student at Lakeside reported being very angry with one of the hospital neurologists because he refused to order a diagnostic test they considered essential.

The details of the case, as it was described by the house officers, went as follows. A woman with a history of tuberculosis and a seizure disorder (which had been successfully controlled for many years by the drugs Dilantin and phenobarbital) had been admitted to the hospital complaining of muscle weakness, and the intern had felt from the start that a muscle biopsy would be the most useful test to determine the nature and cause of her disease. The private family doctor had turned the case over to a neurologist and indicated that he should manage it as he wished. For two weeks the patient was put through a series of diagnostic tests (including various kinds of x-rays: a barium enema, upper GI series, intravenous pyelogram of the renal system, repeated chest films) as well as various laboratory tests (such as Shilling test, sedimentation rate, A.N.A. titer, L.E. prep, Latex Fixation, sma-12, Tensilon test, serum electrophoresis, thyroid studies, and various others).

Despite daily requests in the patient's chart from the intern urging that a muscle biopsy be done (he would repeatedly note: "Plan: Would get a muscle Bx as soon as possible. Would like to proceed with muscle Bx immediately."), the neurologist failed to arrange for such a test. One of the house officers suspected that the neurologist was stalling to use up the maximum two weeks of hospital visiting fees allowed to him by the patient's insurance plan. The intern complained to the family doctor who had referred the case to the neurologist that they were wasting time and money by not doing the muscle biopsy and "going where the money is" (a phrase often used by doctors to indicate the decisive test), but the physician replied that he was pleased with the way the neurologist was handling the case and saw no need to intervene. The intern reported that whenever he tried to reach the neurologist he was told that the neurologist was busy or out of the office, and permission to order the test was refused. Finally, after two weeks the intern complained to the Chief of Medicine, who in turn called up the family doctor to ask why they were delaying. According to the intern, the doctor feigned surprise and exclaimed, "You mean, she hasn't had the muscle biopsy yet?"

The biopsy finally revealed what they had suspected—the patient suffered from an autoimmune syndrome that required that her medication of Dilantin (for her seizures) be discontinued, and that she be placed on a regimen of steroids. However, before they could initiate the steroid treatments, they wanted to be certain that her tuberculosis was no longer present, since steroids could activate a dormant tuberculosis condition, and this required obtaining a series of sputum samples.

The house officers confessed that by this time they were very angry with the neurologist and family physician for keeping them waiting so long for the muscle biopsy. So the house officers, in turn, decided to keep the private doctors waiting for the tuberculosis results. Each morning they would "forget" to obtain the sputum—and since the sputum had to be collected early in the morning before breakfast (and before either of the private doctors was around to check up on the house officers), they kept "finding" it inconvenient to obtain the sample because of other, more pressing duties.

In the meantime, several more days had passed and the patient remained in the hospital, deliberately ignored by the resentful house officers, and having come no closer to starting a treatment. But because her Dilantin had been discontinued, early one morning she suffered from a seizure and fell to the ground. She was found lying on the floor by another patient, who reported that the patient was "confused, stuporous, and foaming at the mouth." When the patient was finally brought out of this condition she was left with a face and scalp so badly bruised that she had to undergo tests for a possible skull fracture. The next day, despite orders that she be confined to bed, she could be seen staggering up and down the hospital corridors with black-and-blue eyes and a badly bruised head.

This illustration is not at all unusual in the sense that house officers and private doctors frequently squabble over tests as a way of exercising control. One intern explained the situation from his point of view (though the private doctor might have disagreed):

"The private doctors will do the same tests on different patients in different ways, just to keep us in the position of having to ask them what they want each and every time. If there are two ways of doing the same thing, call them A and B, then if I suggest doing A on a patient, then the private doctor will say, no, do B. Then on the next patient with the same doctor if I say O.K., we'll do B, then the doc will say, no, do A. They switch around like that each time the same thing comes up so it will be clear that they are in control."

House officers at Lakeside also complained that private doctors would make trivial changes in the orders written by house staff in the charts, simply to remind the house officers that the private doctors were in control. It was commonly joked that if a surgical intern wrote an order in a chart, such as: "Check blood pressure every 30 minutes," the private doctor might cross out the order and write, "Check blood pressure every 20 minutes for the first hour, and then once every 45 minutes thereafter."

Orders and counterorders written in a patient's chart often serve as a subtle or obvious expression of the opinions that doctors hold of one another, and doctors are consequently highly sensitive about changes of orders written into a chart. It is a touchy matter, for the change by one doctor of another doctor's orders may carry with it a show of challenge, criticism or disrespect. In the following incident about a rather significant change in a chart order, we may observe just how far the battle of the charts may go.

Whenever a patient who had ever been under the care of Dr. Maris was admitted to the hospital, it was widely known at Lakeside that the patient was to be admitted to Maris's service (the thoracic service) even if the difficulty had nothing to do with cardiac surgery. Ordinarily, a patient seen in the Emergency Room would be assigned to the service most appropriate for the illness, but Maris maintained that his patients constituted special cases: having had cardiac surgery, they were to be treated as exceptions and all of them were to be admitted as his patients, no matter what the illness. On one occasion, however, a patient who had undergone cardiac surgery under Maris's care some years before was admitted to the hospital's medical service, with a diagnosis of "coronary heart failure." Dr. Maris had nonetheless paid a consulting visit to the patient, and disagreed with the medical diagnosis of CHF, arguing that the patient suffered instead from a surgical condition. His note read: "This pleasant, senile, cachectic man is substantially obstructed by his esophageal stricture, secondary to hiatus hernia. He is not in CHF but rather suffers from volume depletion and should receive fluid and transfusions of whole blood."

After writing the note, Maris notified his house officers to expect a transfer of the man to their thoracic service. But instead of reading and regarding the consulting note as a subtle order to transfer the patient to the thoracic service, the resident instead persisted with his original diagnosis. Underneath the order for the transfusion written by Maris, the resident briefly noted, "Cancel above order," and in his medical note, he disregarded the senior doctor's analysis and remarked: "There has been no urine output. Plan is to continue watching closely re Coronary Heart Failure and urine output. May need diuresis [removal of water] and digoxin. But in a 78-pound 77-year-old man, this could be more trouble than it's worth."

According to the thoracic intern, Maris read the note with shock that a medical resident would question his authority and dismiss his order so casually. Moreover, Maris was convinced that the resident showed remarkable stupidity in coming to such a diagnosis, and he was upset that the standing order, to diurese the patient, would be exactly the opposite of what he felt was needed. Whenever he would pass someone in the hospital corridor that day, Maris would stop them to describe the stupidity of the resident, pointing out that the patient's dry tear ducts obviously indicated that the patient was dehydrated rather than in coronary heart failure. His thoracic intern agreed, adding that the patient looked like a "dried-up prune." Maris told the intern that he was so pleased with the description they would have to include it in their next note in the patient's chart.

As the thoracic intern told the story, Maris spent considerable time that afternoon making phone calls around town trying to obtain the exact wording of a quotation from Shakespeare that he wished to include in his rebuttal note. The following morning Maris entered his note in the chart, partially reproduced below:

> There has been much controversy here about this gentleman, and the proper treatment. In my humble opinion, he is *clearly not* in Coronary Heart Failure because:
> a   The rales in my opinion are due to overflow of secretions from a totally obstructed esophagus. This is quite standard in these situations. I have seen x-rays and they *are not CHF.*
> b   He is obviously volume depleted with desiccated subcutaneous tissue.
> c   He is not in CHF, furthermore, because
> 1   He lies flat without dyspnea [shortness of breath]
> 2   He fills his jugular veins from ↓ not ↑ [above not below]
> 3   His eyeballs are sunken
> 4   He has the appearance of a "prune."
> In short, this patient is volume depleted and needs fluid and whole blood volume expansion. The thought that there is a contraindication to blood transfusion must be qualified in the light of what I consider straightforward indications of need and the lack of danger of transfusions. (One patient met with jaundice in 7,000 transfusions here last year).
>
> P. MARIS.
>
> Addendum: Reading on the subject of dehydration can begin with Shakespeare's death of Falstaff (ca 1599): "for after I saw him fumble with the sheets and play with flowers and smiles upon his fingers' ends, I knew there was but one way; for his nose was sharp as a pen, and a' babbled of green fields."
>
> MARIS.

As Maris signed the note he remarked with satisfaction to

his intern: "They will transfer him to us within an hour, so be ready for him."

As the intern later explained, it was no surprise that they would transfer the old man to the thoracic service. He was no joy to treat, being an old nursing home patient, and the medical resident had already had his fun with the case.

Within the hour, the medical resident noted: "EKG; Ambued; Rales in both sides of lung; Transferred to service of Dr. P. Maris."

PART

II

OVERLOOKING MEDICAL MISTAKES

MEDICAL MISTAKES: An Introduction

EVERY OCCUPATION PRESENTS some special set of risks for the individuals who work at it. Some types of employment, such as police work or fire fighting, carry a significant physical risk. Those who try to create and maintain small businesses are usually taking a significant financial gamble. But every line of work carries its own particular set of psychological, social, financial and physical risks. Work risks are heightened by the fact that almost everyone makes mistakes at some points in his work career, mistakes that may be highly consequential either to the worker himself or to other persons for whom he is in some way responsible.

It is understandable, then, that those who are subject to the same work risks will construct collective rationalizations and defenses to help them through their mistakes and to protect themselves from the reactions of the lay world. For example, if a policeman, in the line of duty, mistakenly draws a gun and shoots an individual who turns out to be unarmed, he is likely to be loyally supported by his fellow policemen. Even if the policeman in question had exercised very poor judgment in firing the shot, his fellow police officers are likely to defend his action as reasonable and justified, because they know that such mistakes could easily happen to any one of them and because they feel that the special risks of their job expose them to difficulties that lay outsiders do not have to face. Indeed, in those lines of work that entail high risks (either for the worker or for the client) the construction of collective justifications for mistakes will occupy an important place in the work experience.

The risks of medical work are very high; mistakes made in the line of duty may cost a human life. While the physician is not subject to physical risk himself, as the policeman is, he *is* subject to the extraordinary feelings of responsibility for damaging a life that has been entrusted to his care. To protect themselves against these feelings, those in the medical profession employ several collective rationales for distancing themselves from the outcomes of their mistakes. Consequently, one could not hope to understand what medical work is about without understanding how the neutralization of mistakes fits into the ideology and organization of medical work. By "neutralization" of medical mistakes I mean the various processes by which medical mistakes are systematically ignored, justified, or made to appear unimportant or inconsequential by the doctors who have made them or those who have noticed that they have been made.

At every stop and turn of medical work, there are built-in professional protections for the doctor against having to recognize and take responsibility for mistakes made on patients. These defenses against acknowledging mistakes reside in the very heart of medical work, philosophy and organization. Furthermore, every aspect of medical work is shaped by this group collusion to ignore and justify errors.

Indeed, the very definition of what constitutes a medical mistake is carefully controlled by doctors. What would probably be viewed as a mistake by the patient may not be interpreted as a mistake by the physician, and the doctor usually has the power to control the identification of mistakes. The definition of mistakes becomes so restrictive in medical practice as to give truth to the statement: "The operation was a success but the patient died," for although it is expressed as a joke by lay persons, this is a statement that has legitimacy in the view of many doctors. Within the professional group, what is seen as a success and what a failure, what is regarded as good or bad medicine, may have little to do with the interests and concerns of the particular patient.

There is a tendency in any line of work (especially those requiring skills acquired in long training) for its practitioners to start to think of the work as an "art" and to evaluate the work more in terms of the creativity or technical brilliance of those who do it than in terms of criteria meaningful or relevant to those who are the recipients of the work or service. Thus, surgery may become an art to those who practice it, and technical mastery may become more important to the "artists" than the practical outcome for particular clients.

Chapter 1, "The Ultimate in Surgery," is an account of a few actual operations and the people involved in them, and illustrates some of the ways that surgeons protect themselves against having to recognize the consequences of what they do to patients: surgeons in these circumstances often attend to the "art" and technical achievement of the work, or to the overall scientific merit of the procedure, rather than to the actual outcome for the individual patient.

Still, even given the very restrictive ideas among doctors about what is a medical mistake, there are times when mistakes are so apparent even to doctors as to demand some sort of collegial reaction. And it is here that doctors develop group techniques for justifying their errors and minimizing the appearance of injury to the patient. A good place to observe this retrospective neutralization and the collective rationalization of mistakes is the Medical Mortality Review Conference (also called Mortality and Morbidity or "M & M" Meeting), for the avowed purpose of these regular hospital meetings is to review cases that ended in a patient death in which there is controversy over the proper treatment and/or a question of medical mismanagement. As the chapter "Mortality Review" illustrates, although the official purpose of these meetings is to serve an educational and regulatory function of detecting mistakes and preventing their recurrence, in fact these meetings often operate in such ways as to justify retrospectively the error and excuse the physician of any blame.

One cannot understand the ways that doctors relate to medical mistakes without taking into account the surrounding context of special loyalties and group affiliations within the hospital. Whether doctors will define an activity as a mistake, and how they will respond to it, depends a great deal upon the operation of conflicting interests and rivalries of different groups of doctors within the hospital. What is considered a mistake by a cardiologist will not be so considered by a surgeon. Furthermore, the right to intervene in another doctor's activities, and the responsibility (or lack of it) for cooperating or even participating in another doctor's error, is determined by the particular configuration of statuses and specialties of the doctors involved. All of this is to say that the ideas, rules, and practices about mistakes among doctors are not determined by any universal standard of right and wrong, or good and bad medical practice, but rather emerge from the practical interests of each department, hierarchical rank, and specialty group as they go about their routine daily work. The influence of special group loyalties on even the definition of mistakes becomes obvious in the chapter on "Mortality Review" as well as in the one that follows. And in many private teaching hospitals, the ambiguity about who has authority and responsibility for regulating the quality of care often allows incompetence to go unchecked.

Finally, it can be safely argued that although doctors may have differences and rivalries among themselves with regard to defining, blaming and acting on mistakes, all doctors will join hands and close ranks against patients and the public. The chapter "Closing the Ranks and Keeping the Patient Uninformed" illustrates how most doctors are willing to forget their differences in order to protect themselves and their common interests against lay outsiders.

The medical mistakes described in these chapters are primarily situations in which the errors were made by private physicians, rather than by the residents or interns. Mistakes of residents and interns are a completely different matter, for making mistakes when one is a house officer is seen as a natural part of the training process. And although residents and interns may be reprimanded for mistakes, they are also seen as working with a "beginner's license" that grants them some pardon from responsibility.

A few more things must be said about the relationship between physician training and the response to mistakes. One of the reasons that many doctors in training feel that they should not be held responsible for mistakes is that they have to learn how to do things, and in medicine it is widely assumed (correctly or not) that the only way to learn medicine is to do it. This means that inexperienced interns and residents are often given great freedom, and indeed are required, to act upon their own judgment, even to the point of being allowed to make serious mistakes. In medical training there is a widely used expression about mastering procedures (such as lumber punctures or inserting an endotracheal tube) which goes: "See one, do one, teach one." The meaning of this remark is that medical students and interns are told very early that they have to pay attention and learn quickly because nobody is going to "hold their hand," and they will have to make decisions and do procedures all by themselves.

Furthermore, they come to believe (realistically or not) that one day they will be in an emergency situation where they will have to do a medical procedure usually done by a specialist (such as a liver biopsy) by themselves, and they had better know how to do it. In reality, most doctors who work in urban medical centers will probably never face such a situation, but it is still felt that they must try these procedures when they can during their training years. Given the "see one, do one, teach one" approach, these procedures are often attempted with little supervision by inexperienced house officers.

Finally, because of the heavily emphasized value of self-sufficiency in medicine, it is very difficult for a doctor (of any rank) to admit that he doesn't know how to do something, or that he needs assistance. This feature of medical work enters into the overall context in which doctors come to rationalize and justify errors, even long after their training is completed.

4

MEDICAL MORTALITY REVIEW:
A Cordial Affair

A MORTALITY AND MORBIDITY conference for doctors bears some resemblance to a wedding or a funeral for members of a family. In all these ceremonies there is some feeling among those who attend that tact and restraint must be exercised if everyone is to leave on friendly terms. But steering a mortality meeting along on a pleasant and even course is occasionally difficult, for as in weddings and funerals, the very nature of the event often prompts participants to come dangerously close to saying to one another those upsetting things that are usually left unsaid.

Mortality meetings are regularly scheduled conferences at Lakeside Hospital; they are held in a large auditorium to accommodate the entire medical staff (private attending physicians, house officers, and teaching staff). Their avowed purpose is to review, in fine detail, those medical cases that ended in an in-hospital patient death, and in which there is some question of error, failure, or general mismanagement on the part of the physicians involved. One of the implicit if unspoken concerns that always underlies the review is the question of whether the patient's death might have been avoided had the medical judgment been more sound, for what is usually involved in these cases is a question of misdiagnosis or of appropriate medical action taken too late.

In consideration of the delicacy of the occasion, the meetings are restricted to the medical staff of the hospital. Even the surgical staff is generally not invited. The surgical service has its own mortality meetings, and a surgeon would be considered meddlesome for attending a medical mortality conference simply out of curiosity. Only those surgeons who were directly involved in a particular case under consideration will be asked to attend a medical mortality meeting. Families are *not* informed that their deceased relative's case has been chosen for review. Although the meetings may be considerably embarrassing for the doctors involved, the Medical Mortality Conference is, at least on the surface, treated as as an *educational* rather than a punitive affair. At Lakeside, the conferences are not investigations or formal hearings held to consider the competence of particular doctors, although they are often presented this way on television medical dramas. There are no formal sanctions applied to doctors at the end of these conferences. Rather, Mortality Review Conferences are "educational" sessions organized around reviewing particular cases rather than individual doctors, even though the cases are selected because there is disagreement over the appropriate treatment and often a question of physician error involved.

The Mortality Review Conference has a special quality of high tension, and the meetings are better attended than are those of the other regular teaching conferences. At Lakeside Hospital, the Chief of Medicine stands on the stage and presides over the Mortality Review Conference as a master of ceremonies. As the case is reviewed in chronological order, starting with the time of the patient admission to the hospital, and proceeding to the autopsy report, the chief calls on the various doctors who were involved in the case, asks them to step to the front of the auditorium, and instructs them to recall and explain what they did and what they thought at each moment in time. He counsels them not to jump ahead of the chronological order, nor to divulge information gained at a later time, in order not to spoil the final diagnosis for the members of the audience. As one after another of the staff testifies about how they were led to the same mistaken diagnosis, a convincing case for the justifiability of the error is implicitly presented and the responsibility for the mistake is spread so that no one doctor is made to look guilty of a mistake that anyone else wouldn't have made, and in fact, didn't make. As in a good detective story, the case is reconstructed to show that there was evidence for suspecting an outcome different from the one that turns out to be the true circumstance. Responsibility for the error is also neutralized by making much of unusual or misleading features of the case, or showing how the patient was himself to blame, because of uncooperative or neurotic behavior. Furthermore, by reviewing the case in fine detail the doctors restore their images as careful, methodical practitioners and thereby neutralize the actual sloppiness and carelessness made obvious by the mistake. The doctors' discomfort is further minimized by treating the review as an educational occasion rather than an investigatory event.

In order to appreciate the special atmosphere and significance of the Mortality Review, it is important to understand that doctors who work together ordinarily live by a gentlemen's agreement to overlook each other's mistakes. The aim is not merely to hide errors and incompetence from the patients and the public, but also to avoid interfering in one another's work and to avoid acknowledgment of the injury that has been done to patients. Such a conspiracy to look the other way regarding the failures of one's colleagues is not always recognized by the doctors for what it is, for a blindness to injury done to patients and a convincing set of justifications and excuses for medical mistakes are carefully built into their training and professional etiquette. Most doctors are therefore capable of comfortably viewing themselves as altruistic and highly responsible practitioners all the while they engage in collective rationalizations for ignoring and condoning each other's errors and incompetence.

Still, there are special occasions in the hospital routine, such as the Mortality Meeting, when doctors are gathered together to examine the sorts of unpleasant facts they would otherwise ignore. At these times a great deal of effort is expended to make the embarrassing facts seem less damaging. For if such medical incompetence or error were fully and publicly (among themselves) acknowledged, physician-colleagues might feel forced to take measures against one another, and this is one of the things they least like to do.

As the Chief of Medicine at Lakeside explained, "Eighty percent of the mistakes made around here are ignored or swept under the rug. I can only pick *certain* cases for mortality review—it's got to be a cordial affair."

Perhaps that description of the selection procedures for mortality review accounts for the curious fact that at Lakeside, most of the medical situations presented at these conferences conveniently seem to involve an illness that would have ended in the patient's death in any case, even if the correct diagnosis had been made immediately. There is a strange absence of cases reviewed in these meetings in which the patient would clearly have lived had it not been for the medical mismanagement. By selecting only those cases in which the physician's error was not fateful in an ultimate sense the discussion of mistakes largely becomes an academic affair.

Practicality rather than sentiment is the key to the tact and reserve with which doctors respond to each other's errors. A doctor's reluctance to criticize a colleague's mistakes to his face at a large meeting is not motivated out of respect or affection. Indeed, many doctors are willing, in small groups, to say that another physician (not present) is a menace or a terrible doctor. And even at the mortality review conferences, those doctors who are not involved in a case may occasionally sit back and enjoy the gentle roasting of a disliked work associate. The reluctance to point out and criticize another doctor's mistakes at an official meeting comes rather out of a fear of reprisal and a recognition of common interests. For each doctor knows that he has made some more or less terrible mistake in his career, and that he is likely to make others— mistakes, moreover, which will be obvious to his colleagues. That is why, in matters of peer regulation, doctors observe the Golden Rule.

So it is that mortality meetings are built upon a simultaneous admission and cover-up of mistakes. For although the avowed purpose of these meetings is to review mistakes and prevent their recurrence, in actuality the meetings are organized and conducted in ways that absolve the doctors from responsibility and guilt and provide the self-assuring but somewhat false appearance that physicians are monitoring each other and their standards of work. In case after case physician errors are systematically excused and justified, and their consequences made to look unimportant.

Before turning to some actual cases, it should be noted that despite the tact and sensitivity with which doctors treat each other's errors, a mortality meeting is not an entirely comfortable situation. Like a family trying collectively to ignore that the father is having an affair, or that the daughter is a drug addict, the doctors at a mortality meeting are often pushed to extreme displays of courtesy to overlook the worst and find good excuses for regrettable behavior.

CASE NO. 1: JONATHAN THOMAS

Jonathan Thomas was a thirty-four-year-old insurance salesman who had complained of abdominal pain and black stool (indicating gastrointestinal bleeding). His problem was diagnosed as a gastric ulcer and he was placed on a regimen of tranquilizers and an ulcer diet. His subsequent complaints were explained as being consistent with an ulcer and a neurotic personality. Ten months later Jonathan Thomas died of cancer spread throughout his abdominal cavity.

This was to be a particularly uncomfortable case for the staff to consider in Mortality Review because of a number of factors. First of all, the patient was a young man with a large family, and this made his life more valuable in the eyes of the doctors. Second, mistakes in diagnosis had been made repeatedly, and important information overlooked more than once. Third, a large number of people had been involved in this case, and while this offered the consolation of spreading out the responsibility, it also pointed out the weaknesses of the hospital consulting system. For if not one of a dozen physicians had caught the obvious errors, it was probably because each of the consultants involved in the case had been too accepting of each other's erroneous assumptions instead of carefully doing the diagnostic jobs they were supposed to be doing.

Notices about the mortality meeting had been distributed days beforehand and signs posted around the hospital. The chief's secretary had made sure that all the doctors involved in the case would be there for the review. As always, the meeting was held in the large theaterlike auditorium and members of the staff seated themselves in the rows of seats facing the stage in a steep incline.

The meeting was called to order by the Chief of Medicine, who welcomed everyone and made brief announcements of unrelated matters. Next, an intern described the hospital's mortality profile for the preceding month: he described how many patients had died in the hospital in each major disease category. Finally, the Chief of Medicine, Dr. Tanner, returned to the stage and introduced the Thomas case. As usual, the patient's history was reviewed in chronological order, each doctor being called to the front of the room to recall his thoughts and describe his participation at that moment in time in the case.

The early history was reviewed by Dr. Backman, the specialist in gastrointestinal disorders who had managed the case. Backman was highly respected and well-liked by most of the staff, and so there were no undertones of questioning his competence but rather friendly empathy for the usually careful physician who had made an uncharacteristic mistake. From the beginning, Backman explained, he had assumed that the gastrointestinal bleeding indicated by the black stool was caused by a stress-induced gastric ulcer: "What led us down the garden path last October was the fact that he was taking on added responsibility for his family's business. The sudden pain seemed to coincide with that, so we put him on an ulcer regimen and gave him tranquilizers and released him in satisfactory condition. After discharge, a GI series was negative, but epigastric pain reappeared and in April he reported severe upper left quadrant pains which became persistent."

Dr. Jenkins, one of the supervisors of the teaching program, interrupted: "Was this severe upper left quadrant pain different from the epigastric pain? Was it something new?"

Dr. Backman: "He described it as different. He had it at night, and it wasn't relieved with antacids."

Dr. Jenkins: "Well, didn't that make you uncomfortable with the diagnosis of gastric ulcer?"

Dr. Backman: "No, because he had resumed smoking and drinking now, and we suspected alcoholic hepatitis, because of his abnormal liver function test. He reported clay-colored stools and we readmitted him to the hospital. From the start of his admission he was quite agitated and needed more sedation, so we called in Dr. Sheingold [the Chief of Psychiatry]."

Dr. Sheingold had considered saying something about Dr. Backman's description of the patient as "drinking again." In fact, he knew the patient drank very little, only a few beers when he went bowling once a week, and it seemed unfair to imply that the man was drinking enough to justify a diagnosis of alcoholic hepatitis. The trouble, Sheingold felt, was that once the doctors decided to bring a psychiatrist into the case most of them no longer believed anything the patient said. And so it had been easy for the doctors to regard this patient as an alcoholic. Still, Dr. Sheingold had observed that Backman was one of the few doctors in the hospital who thought that psychiatry had anything to offer them in their treatment of medical patients, so he had refrained from objecting to the imputation of alcoholism.

Sheingold was motioned to the stage to report on his participation in the case. He began: "Yes, I was invited to walk down the garden path with the others. I talked with the patient on his fourth day of admission. His father-in-law had just retired and appointed the patient as director of the family insurance business. Mr. Thomas had never liked the business and found it morbid. Indeed, he had complicated feelings about his business exacerbated by a long history of depression. Ten years ago he had been responsible for an automobile accident in which his oldest daughter, then three years old, had died. So I was quite sure along with Dr. Backman that this was gastric ulcer disease, and I wrote that in my notes. I also noted that there was an unlikely chance of pancreatic carcinoma [cancer] because I knew that would be considered at some time, but I was quite sure that it was an ulcer."

Dr. Stevens, one of the department chiefs in medicine, had been upset with the reasoning in this case. As he explained, one of his pet peeves was the stupid use of psychiatry, especially by the GI doctors, and he had noticed that Backman was one of the frequent offenders in this regard because as a GI specialist Backman also considered himself something of an expert in the field of psychiatry. As Stevens described the situation, every time one of the GI doctors heard a patient complaint that couldn't be explained he called in a psychiatrist. Stevens wished they would instead just admit to the patient that they didn't know what was wrong, and explain that they would have to wait or do more tests. Instead, complained Stevens, a psychiatrist came in and spoke to the patient and *always* found a psychiatric complication. "And," concluded Stevens, "what did that tell you? That everyone has problems?"

Dr. Rosen, another internist on the hospital staff, was questioning Backman. "Why weren't the clay-colored stools considered? Didn't you believe him?"

Backman replied: "Well, the clay-colored stools could have been caused by the antacids he was taking, but to be perfectly frank, I didn't know how much credence I could give to his reports. He was quite upset and had gone into a rage about having to pay for the use of the television in his room. I should also add that he was now complaining about leg pain as well. He was re-endoscoped and a liver scan was taken. It showed an enlarged liver without focal abnormalities and the liver function was not impaired. A liver biopsy was normal, which surprised us. We expected to find alcoholic hepatitis. After the biopsy there was hemoptysis (coughing up blood). We were concerned because that had never happened and we thought that bleeding from the liver biopsy might have gone into the lung area. We did a cholangiogram and it was normal, but we noted that he had an elevated alkaphosphotase level. We released him from the hospital once again on a bland diet with tranquilizers, and his discharge diagnosis was peptic ulcer."

Dr. Davis, one of the younger internists, directed more questions to Backman: "Why wasn't a surgical exploration done at this time?"

Backman smiled, shaking his head. "I'm not sure. I guess we weren't smart enough." Davis continued: "Why was no attention paid to the calf pain?" Backman answered: "The reason we ignored his complaints of leg pain was that his roommate in the hospital had thrombophlebitis in the leg. So when Thomas complained of it, it just seemed too coincidental and we figured it was just a hysterical reaction."

Dr. Sheingold was afraid that this case was certainly not going to encourage the doctors in the hospital to turn to the psychiatry department for help. It made him angry that the only situation in which most of the doctors considered psychiatry to be useful was for the management of what they considered a "crazy" patient, and once a patient in the hospital was seen by a psychiatrist the doctors would attribute to the patient all sorts of psychological mechanisms that had nothing to do with the patient's personality (in this case they were imputing "hysterical" behavior to a non-hysterical patient) and they wouldn't even read the notes that Sheingold wrote in the patient's chart about which psychological mechanisms were relevant. Also, since they didn't regard psychiatric illness as real, they always disliked patients with psychiatric symptoms. As Sheingold later explained, all the doctors had disliked this patient when they thought that he suffered only from an ulcer, and they had only decided that he was likable after they realized that he was "really" sick with cancer.

Backman was still explaining why he had released the

patient despite abnormal laboratory findings. "Oh, and to finish your question about surgery—his abdominal pains went away after three days, so we didn't consider it any more." He leafed through the pages of the chart and continued. "He was readmitted the following week with a swollen foot, an enlarged liver, extensive thrombophlebitis." Backman nodded to Cohen, the cardiologist who had been consulted at this point. Cohen stood up and briefly spoke from his place in the audience. "I was asked to say whether the problem was due to pulmonary emboli or from hemoptysis to the lung from the liver biopsy. I thought he had pulmonary emboli."

Attention was now directed to the Chief of Surgery, who described his part in the case: "I saw him at this point and I knew something terrible was going on. He was going downhill rapidly. It looked like an abdominal mass. The plan was now to deal with his phlebitis—so here we were in a bind. We had a GI bleeder who had to be anticoagulated for his emboli [a treatment that would increase bleeding], and now he had shortness of breath. The problem in dealing with this patient was that he was dead opposed to surgery. He had been in the life insurance business all his life, and every time we talked about surgery he would say, 'Now my family's gonna be collecting on my policy.'" The surgeon turned to Davis, who had earlier criticized Backman for not calling in a surgeon sooner. "I'll tell you why we didn't do an exploratory laparotomy [surgical investigation] earlier. He was so frantic and had been sick so long. He had abdominal pain, and calf pain and GI bleeding. He dreaded surgery, and frankly I dreaded going in there. His wife kept yelling at me, asking what was wrong, and when I said I didn't know she called me stupid. I guess maybe we *were* stupid. Anyway that's why we didn't do an exploratory earlier." In the back of the auditorium, some of the medical residents were smiling and mumbling that the reason the Chief had delayed surgery was that he hated to operate. Douglas had a reputation among the younger aggressive doctors in the hospital of being too cautious and slow to act. It was not clear whether Douglas noticed their remarks, and he continued. "So we did a venous clip and when we later did an exploratory we saw that there was cancer all over. The patient died three days later, and I just want to add here that according to the chart he was in severe anguish on the last day of his life, and was not given the pain-killers we had prescribed, so we can thank our nurses for making the last day of his life as miserable as possible." The surgeon nodded to the pathologist and the lights were switched off. Color slides of the patient's affected organs were flashed on the screen. Each one showed gross abnormalities from the spread of the cancer. Throughout the auditorium murmurs could be heard at the extensiveness of the cancer, as if to emphasize that with so dramatic and pervasive a disease they as doctors could hardly have been expected to stop such an invasion.

When the lights were turned on the surgeon drew the meeting to a close, explaining how at that very moment the patient's brother was waiting in his office; the brother had come to show him an article about a so-called wonder drug, which was illegal, for curing cancer. Douglas added that he had given the brother an appointment so that the man could yell at him for having refused to try this illegal drug. Several doctors in the audience laughed and shook their heads sympathetically, breaking into small groups as they moved into the adjoining room for coffee and doughnuts.

The Thomas case, described above, illustrates how doctors often justify their errors by pointing to misleading or unusual features of the case. By demonstrating that they had good reason (though later shown to be mistaken) for doing what they did, they may avoid censure and discomfort, and save face before their colleagues. Physical symptoms inconsistent with the final diagnosis are the misleading cues which provide the most comforting and persuasive type of excuse for making the wrong diagnosis. However, when physical justifications are unavailable, doctors often resort to psychological and social evidence as the factors which misguided them and justified their behavior. In these cases, the nonphysical evidence is represented as being so convincing as to justify overlooking even physical evidence which should have alerted doctors to the correct diagnosis. In the Thomas case, for example, the doctors overlooked clear symptoms of organic disorder (such as the elevated alkaphosphotase level) because they were so convinced that the patient was neurotic and that his complaints and symptoms could be explained psychologically.

In other cases where physical findings are overlooked, or erroneously discounted, the physician will often excuse his embarrassing error by blaming the patient. If the patient can be "discredited" as crazy, alcoholic, obnoxious, uncooperative, or otherwise difficult or undeserving, then the responsibility for the medical error can be shifted away from the doctor to the patient. The physician's errors are made to seem understandable and inconsequential in a life fated for disaster by the patient's own doing. The following case illustrates this process.

CASE NO. 2: ALICE MC DONALD

Mrs. McDonald was a fifty-year-old woman who died in the Emergency Room of a perforated duodenal ulcer which the staff failed to diagnose, despite her complaints of severe abdominal pain.

The case was introduced in the meeting by the intern who had seen her in the Emergency Room. He opened the discussion by describing her as "An obese, alcoholic woman of Irish extraction who was very uncooperative and used very abusive language," thereby fixing her in the minds of the physicians in the audience as the type of patient who is difficult to treat.

In explaining why they had not paid much attention to her complaints of abdominal pain, the doctors involved in the case made much of her appearance of being "mentally disconnected." Asked to be more specific about her mental state, both the intern and the medical doctor covering the Emergency Room that night stated that they remembered noting the smell of alcohol on her breath, and therefore felt they could dismiss her complaints as the ravings of a drunken woman.

Toward the end of the meeting someone in the audience offhandedly asked what the alcohol level in the blood had been at the time of the incident. Now the Chief of Medicine sheepishly admitted a fact that had been previously left unmentioned: although much had been made of this woman's drunkenness, the fact was that the alcohol level in the blood had been zero at the time of her examination.

This embarrassing fact was passed over quickly. No longer able to use her drunkenness as an excuse for their failure to take her complaints seriously, the doctors now turned more exclusively to emphasizing her angry, "disconnected" and uncooperative behavior toward them as the factor responsible for the poor treatment she received.

The power of the doctor's self-justification is highlighted in this case. For even after implicitly acknowledging that drunkenness was falsely attributed to the patient, the doctors continued to blame this woman's death on her own anger and abusive language, and ignored the possibility that such behavior was appropriate for a woman dying in great pain while the doctors around her treated her complaints as the fabrications of a hysterical alcoholic.

The case also illustrates how doctors may overlook important physical findings (which should indicate a serious illness) if they have already discounted the complaints by viewing the patient as a certain kind of neurotic individual. For a "neurotic" individual is viewed by doctors as an unreliable reporter, and once characterized this way, a patient's remarks are likely to be ignored. Indeed, these patients are commonly known among many doctors as "crocks" or "turkeys" and are considered undeserving of serious attention.

It is a complicated problem, for certainly doctors will

occasionally meet with an anxious patient who will refuse to believe that he is in good health. But serious errors are often made as a result of characterizing patients as "crocks," for doctors are usually not in a position to correctly guess who is really sick and who isn't, from behavior alone. Furthermore, doctors appear to assign the label "crock" quite often on grounds of personal or prejudiced responses. They are more likely, for example, to dismiss a patient as neurotic and not really sick if the patient seems angry, mistrustful, or disrespectful to the doctor (as we shall see in Chapter 9). The label "crock" also seems to be applied erroneously more often to women.

A third case reviewed in the Medical Mortality Conference illustrates another common pattern in neutralizing mistakes. Sometimes the patient may be viewed as so lacking in social value or otherwise so physically deteriorated that the question of a consequential medical mistake hardly occurs to anyone involved in the case. That is, the recognition of, and attention to, a medical mistake depends upon the doctor's seeing the patient as an individual having some value. The very definition of a mistake, by doctors, therefore, rests not on some universal and fixed standard of good or poor practice applied to every case, but the definition of a mistake rather shifts and slides according to the value of the patient as assessed by the doctors.

As this final Mortality Review case illustrates, the patient was viewed as so physically and socially worthless that the audience paid little attention to the one doctor among them who expressed distress at how the case had been handled.

CASE NO. 3: FREDDY GRAZZO

Freddy Grazzo had become a well-known patient in Lakeside Hospital, and his case the source of many jokes among the staff. He was a clear example of what many physicians think of as the "garbage" or deadwood of their work and clientele. Elderly, unmarried and unemployed, Freddy Grazzo lived in a rooming house and spent his days drinking beer with his friends. He had an undiagnosed illness that repeatedly brought him to the Emergency Room, close to death and in pulmonary edema (his lungs filled with fluid, and breathing with great difficulty). Each time, the resident or intern on duty would resuscitate him and have to do a "work-up" examination as part of the hospital admission. Within a day or two, "Freddy" (as he was called by doctors thirty years his junior) would be doing well enough to leave the hospital, but his furlough was always short: within a few days he would be back in the Emergency Room in the same condition.

Because of his surprising ability to survive one after another of these emergencies Freddy had acquired a wide reputation in the hospital. Any one of these attacks might have ended his life, so it had become something of a standing hospital joke when his emergency admissions began to number in the twenties. Word would spread in the hospital that Freddy was back, and the interns and residents would laugh bitterly about how they had to waste their fine talents on old broken men who would never get better.

Still, over the course of twenty-five admissions a bit of abstract affection for Freddy Grazzo had developed among the staff. As he would be rushed into the Emergency Room, gasping for air, the nurses would tease him that he should be fixed up with Mary O'Leary, who was the female record-breaking survivor of Emergency Room resuscitations. At daily reports to the Chief of Medicine the residents would describe his condition as the "paddle syndrome": like a ball attached to a paddle, he was released from the hospital, went down the street to the nearest bar and soon bounced back into the hospital again.

If the annoyance that the staff felt for this patient were weighed against the amusement, it would have to be said that annoyance prevailed. When Freddy Grazzo arrived in the Emergency Room for the twenty-third time, the charge nurse openly complained that "they shouldn't have even coded him the last time he came in." When patients have an illness that will never improve and when their continued existence seems unwarranted in the doctors' eyes, either the doctor will note in the chart that the patient should not be resuscitated, or word will get passed informally around the staff that the patient should not again be coded the next time he gets into a life-threatening situation.

There was some feeling in the hospital that Freddy Grazzo had already been granted or burdened with too many codes, but he was still to survive this twenty-third admission. As the interns leisurely carried out the resuscitation like a familiar routine and inserted intravenous lines for his drugs, they argued about which floor of the hospital Freddy should be admitted to because no one wanted to do the work-up examination. It was late at night, and when Dr. Jenkins (a physician covering for Dr. Rosen, who was the regular doctor on the case) arrived in the Emergency Room, the charge nurse asked why he had bothered to come in. Jenkins replied that a decision might have to be made that night about keeping the patient alive. (As he put it: "In case something brews tonight a decision should be made.") Although Freddy Grazzo survived this admission, it was not long after that he was one day declared dead on arrival in the Emergency Room.

But even after his death Freddy Grazzo's name was still often heard, because toward the end of his life his physician became convinced that this was no ordinary case of geriatric decline, no mere piece of "medical garbage" after all. Dr. Rosen felt that he might just have stumbled across an exciting rare disease in Freddy Grazzo.

When the mortality meeting was held a few weeks later, Rosen seemed pleased that the case would be reviewed. He had indicated that he was convinced that Freddy had been an unsalvageable patient and he was happy to have a chance to show off his unusual diagnosis.

Rosen had first come to the hospital as a specialist in internal medicine twenty years before. In the old days he had been considered one of the more highly trained physicians in the hospital, and he had been given a free hand in treating the whole range of medical cases, including the most esoteric ones. But in the last few years the power in the hospital had progressively shifted to the newer "subspecialists" on the staff. Now the most challenging heart cases were referred to the cardiologists, and not to doctors like Rosen.

Furthermore, all the internists (an internist is a specialist in internal medicine, not to be confused with an intern, who is an untrained doctor fresh out of medical school) like himself were now expected to call in the specialists for consultations and special diagnostic tests whenever they had anything but the most routine cases. This meant that the specialists wound up managing all the interesting cases while Rosen was supposed to be satisfied with what he called the "lumps and bumps."

His reluctance to bow to pressure and invite consultation from the experts was not a matter of resentment, Rosen had argued to the house officers. For he believed that most consultation from these subspecialists was pointless because their recommendations were completely predictable. For example, during the previous week one of his patients had been admitted after being found unconscious with symptoms possibly suggesting a subarachnoid (brain) hemorrhage. This diagnosis could only have been positively confirmed by doing a somewhat risky and uncomfortable procedure, a cerebral arteriogram. The resident assigned to the case had been in favor of having the diagnostic procedure done, and knowing that Rosen was opposed to it, he had tactfully asked Rosen if they could get a specialist's opinion before ruling it out. Rosen had refused and explained why it was pointless: he could tell the resident exactly what the consultants would say without bothering to have them look at the patient. If the hospital neurologist (who was known to be conservative) was consulted, he would say, "Don't do anything." And if instead, they invited the opinion of the neurosurgeon, he would be sure to say, "Let's operate." So, as Rosen had argued to the resident, since it was all an arbitrary choice, it was better made by the doctor who knew something about the patient (and Rosen felt she was a nervous woman who would be upset by the diagnostic procedure) than on the basis of the prejudice of either subspecialist.

But to return to the Grazzo case, Rosen had indicated his confidence in the care the patient had received, and he was looking forward to the Mortality Review. In fact, he had asked the Chief of Medicine to let him use the entire meeting for this case, although it was customary to go through two cases in each meeting. The chief had refused but compromised by curtailing the discussion on the first case, explaining to the group that he wanted to leave more time for "Hal Rosen's masterpiece."

As Rosen came cheerfully tripping down the stairs to the front of the auditorium he conceded that the case was perhaps a "masterpiece with flaws." Proudly pointing to the twelve volumes of the patient's chart, he apologized that because of time constraints they would have to begin their review with the patient's eighteenth hospital admission. The facts were as follows: the patient had suffered recurrent dyspnea (breathlessness) and pulmonary edema, would often faint after eating, and they had long suspected that the cause of the symptoms were pulmonary emboli which were causing the edema. To illustrate the symptoms, Rosen entertained the audience with stories of how Freddy Grazzo would collapse on the street but somehow always get to the hospital in time to be resuscitated. On one occasion, Rosen smiled, Grazzo had suffered a coronary arrest (they believed an embolus had triggered a cardiac arrhythmia) on a street corner in the next town, and he would never have made it to the hospital in time had he not unknowingly reached out and grabbed on to what turned out to be a fire alarm box to steady himself before he collapsed to the ground. A fire truck had arrived within two minutes, and seeing the man collapsed to the ground, the firemen had thrown him on the back of the truck and hauled him into the hospital.

After the laughter subsided Rosen described how they had

made their discovery of the suspected rare disease. One day, upon being released from the hospital, Freddy had been waiting in front of the hospital for a taxi to take him home only to collapse, once more, into the arms of Rosen's colleague, Dr. Paul Jenkins, who had been walking by. Grabbing him in his arms, Jenkins had suddenly had the inspiration that the patient might be suffering not from pulmonary emboli but rather from the interesting and unusual central nervous hyperventilation syndrome. And, Rosen concluded with a smile, he concurred.

What followed next was some friendly joking about whether Rosen was only daydreaming to come up with such a diagnosis. Gordon Frank, the Chief of Cardiology, looked annoyed and finally openly expressed his disapproval. Standing up, he interrupted the friendly teasing: "I am deeply disturbed by the levity of this meeting, and I must say it matches the levity with which this patient was admitted every time to the Coronary Care Unit. Each time he came in everyone would giggle 'Guess who's back, ha-ha.' And I think that instead of sending him into our unit each time without knowing what was wrong with him, the patient should have had tests to ascertain what was wrong. The tests might have shown that he had a treatable illness."

As Frank explained, by saying "I don't like the levity with which this case was handled" he was actually saying that he didn't like the way that Rosen had managed the case medically. There had long been tension and disagreement between Rosen and himself. As he described it, Rosen would never come to him for help when he was out of his depth, and so Frank considered Rosen to be a potentially dangerous doctor. But, he admitted, a doctor couldn't come right out at a Mortality Meeting and say that he didn't like the way someone managed a case, so he had criticized the joking. Those who knew how he felt about Rosen would understand the deeper meaning of his remarks, and those who didn't, or who refused to acknowledge the issue, would be spared an unpleasant scene.

At the Mortality Meeting, Rosen met Frank's challenge and defended his refusal to do the diagnostic tests. There would have been no point, he argued, in performing angiography on this patient because even if the test had shown emboli as the cause of edema, the patient would never have consented to corrective surgery anyway. Frank replied, with obvious irritation, that if Rosen had allowed him to perform a diagnostic angiogram, it might have confirmed one of two possible diseases which were treatable even without surgery. He then described some new procedures, unknown to Rosen, which might have allowed them to treat Grazzo's problem without surgery.

The meeting time was coming to an end and so the doctors in the audience called out their final guesses about the true cause of Freddy Grazzo's illness. The intern who had pronounced the patient dead in the Emergency Room placed his bet on aspiration as the cause of death. An older physician in the audience hazarded the guess of atrial myxoma (a tumor in the heart).

The positions having been staked, it was now time for the final verdict. Solemnly, the pathologist stepped to the front of the room to announce what he had found in his autopsy.

To fully appreciate this moment it must be understood that the part of their work that medical doctors enjoy most is the challenging diagnosis. For most surgeons, the excitement and pleasure in the work is in doing a good job in the operating room: it is in the operating room that surgeons get to use their most highly specialized skills. But for medical doctors, the most exciting opportunity in the work is to make a brilliant diagnosis. Surgeons may also enjoy witnessing a dramatic cure as a result of an operation, but a medical doctor is often denied the satisfaction of bringing about a dramatic cure, especially in the treatment of elderly or chronically ill patients. In such cases, the work of internists can only prolong a painful and limited life. Under these circumstances, pleasure and excitement in the work are found, not in what can be done for patients, but rather in being the first one to come up with a brilliant diagnosis. That is why there would be special satisfaction in turning a routine and boring medical case into a good detective story with a surprising turn of events.

The pathologist, who paused before giving the final verdict on the Grazzo case, did not give away the ending all at once. Instead, he eliminated the losing guesses first. Like runners-up at a beauty contest, those who had guessed incorrectly bowed out good-naturedly. No, the death had not been caused by aspiration; the intern who guessed this possibility received the thumbs-down sign from the doctors sitting around him. And no, there had been no myxoma; the older physician who had made that guess shrugged his shoulders in concession. The pathologist turned to Rosen, sympathetically. While there *had* been some reason to suspect central nervous hyperventilation syndrome, not all of the criteria necessary to make that diagnosis were met in this case, and so that rare disorder could not be claimed. Freddy Grazzo had died the most ordinary death after all: his cardiac arrhythmias (irregularities of the heart beat) had been brought on by atherosclerosis (thickening and occlusion of the walls of the coronary arteries), and it was this common condition of the elderly which had triggered the emboli and his pulmonary edema.

As the meeting broke up, several of Rosen's friends patted him on the back for making a valiant effort at finding an exciting disease.

It is difficult to talk about mistakes without thinking about the feelings which mistakes arouse, both in the individual who has made the error and in the others around him. Acknowledging a consequential mistake is a profoundly upsetting experience for many reasons. First, there is the pain of fully knowing that things might have turned out better had one acted the way one should have. Then there is the unbearable self-doubt that follows from admitting to a mistake. The person who has recognized that he is capable of grave errors is suddenly unable to trust his own judgment. Every future act is cast in doubt and every decision agonized over lest it lead to further disaster. Finally, there is the fact, fair or not, that the individual who has made a mistake is somewhat tarnished in the eyes of his associates, and may even be formally punished or sanctioned. There is sad irony here, for the designation "mistake" is meant, at least on the surface, to excuse or pardon the actor. To say "it was just a mistake" signifies that such a wrong act was out of keeping for such an ordinarily trustworthy individual, just a fluke of nature unlikely to happen again. Nevertheless, most people are naturally suspicious of "mistakes," and the reputation of the person who makes them is often permanently stained.

No wonder, then, that most people try to avoid admitting to mistakes and prefer to live with the continued bad consequences of errors than with the distress of admitting to the mistake. But even if an individual is personally prepared to admit to a mistake, those whose lives and fates are tied up with his own are very likely to talk him out of such an admission, for the acknowledgment of a mistake is upsetting for groups as well as for individuals. When one member of a group starts calling attention to mistakes, not only does everyone else become vulnerable to the same exposure, but the entire collective enterprise they have committed themselves to begins to look more and more shabby.

Groups of doctors are not exempt from the upsetting possibility of having mistakes exposed. The words of just one outspoken member are enough to make everyone uncomfortable. The admission of mistakes is especially upsetting in the world of medicine because it is a world that rests and depends upon a faith in science, objectivity and rationality. A mistake in such a world is as disruptive as the commission of a sin in a religious society. It challenges the most cherished beliefs and identities of its members. Furthermore, since self-sufficiency and self-confidence are so highly valued in the medical profession, an admission of uncertainty or error exposes the physician to the kind of self-doubt that is unacceptable among his colleagues. The admission of a mistake is also very difficult in medicine because the stakes are so high. Many doctors, for example, retain disturbing memories for the rest of their lives of how they were responsible for a patient's death when they were residents because they had been too inexperienced to handle a situation properly.

For all of these reasons, it is not surprising that individual doctors are strictly discouraged by their group and their profession from being too willing to point out a mistake, or to openly admit to a feeling of guilt. The likelihood of making a bad mistake is too high and the price of admitting to it too costly to the group to leave the matter open to the discretion and dispositions of individual members. That is why a doctor is carefully taught in training and afterward not to regard as a mistake what most lay people would consider a mistake, and not to make too much of these unfortunate episodes.

A similar point can be made about feelings of guilt in medicine. Given the probability of making a bad mistake sometime in one's career, and given the probability of recognizing that the cynical reality of medical work is dramatically different from the idealistic expectations and self-images that one began with as a young student, the potential for feeling guilty is very high for physicians. That is why there are strong professional and institutional supports for avoiding feelings of guilt. Indeed, if a doctor is still prone to feeling guilty despite all of the supports to the contrary, he will quickly learn to keep his feelings to himself. Nobody wants to hear about a colleague's feelings of guilt, and talking too freely about such feelings with other doctors is considered a very embarrassing faux pas.

So it is that doctors are not likely to dig too deeply into one another's errors nor even to recognize fully the extent to which they collude in covering up each other's mistakes and incompetence. It is easier for them to shift the blame and responsibility for mistakes away from themselves, either to the patient, who becomes discredited in the process, or to surrounding impersonal circumstances such as misleading or unusual evidence in a particular case. Under these circumstances, mistakes are allowed to flourish and be repeated, and incompetence goes unchecked. Clearly it is the patient who pays the highest price in this arrangement for insuring the comfort of physician-colleagues, but some unusually conscientious doctors also pay the smaller price of being left alone with the residual feelings that manage to survive the professional neutralization and justifications.

5

I JUST WORK HERE: Excuses for Not Intervening in Physician Incompetence

SEVERAL STAFF MEMBERS at Lakeside were surprised when Dr. Bush admitted an eight-year-old girl to the hospital for cardiac surgery. Children who needed cardiac surgery were generally referred to the city's Children's Hospital, which had a large staff that specialized in pediatric cardiac surgery. For cardiac surgery for children is very different from cardiac surgery for adults: it involves very different kinds of cardiac abnormalities, procedures, equipment and surgical considerations. Furthermore, Dr. Bush had not done that much pediatric cardiac surgery in recent years. His experience was primarily limited to the kinds of cardiac surgery most often done on adults with acquired heart disease: valve replacements, pacemaker insertions, and revascularization or bypass procedures. As one of the anesthesiologists pointed out, Bush had not had much recent experience repairing congenital (from birth) cardiac abnormalities in children, and moreover, Lakeside Hospital was not equipped with special pediatric equipment for cardiac surgery. At Lakeside, the child would have to undergo the operation with equipment that had been designed for adult-sized bodies, and without benefit of a team experienced in pediatric procedures and care. Some of the staff who were aware of the situation felt that the child would do much better at the nearby hospital that specialized in pediatric cardiac surgery, but it was not their decision to make.

The child's disease had been diagnosed as an atrial-septal defect (an abnormal hole or opening between the walls of the heart chambers) which had to be repaired and closed. Such a defect is one of the more common congenital abnormalities, and ordinarily not very difficult to repair, so Bush and his assistants had apparently decided that it was reasonable to do the procedure themselves.

Such a situation raises an interesting issue about professional regulation, or the lack of it, in medical practice. It is the informal convention in surgery that a surgeon should not attempt to do procedures at which he is not experienced. When he encounters an esoteric surgical situation that he is not experienced at handling, it is generally believed among doctors that he is ethically bound to refer the patient to someone experienced in that procedure. Naturally, that expectation is especially applicable in situations such as the one described above, where the surgeon knew the situation before the operation, and where there was no emergency, but instead, more than adequate time to make the appropriate referral. Such a rule is actually "informal," however, for as long as a surgeon has operating room privileges in a hospital, he may do whatever he pleases, including procedures at which he is inexperienced.

But despite the general belief among doctors that surgeons should refer esoteric cases to specialists, there is also a counter-expectation in the world of surgery which says that a good surgeon should be able to stand up to and face any unexpected situation without backing down or needing help, simply by keeping cool and using his intelligence and knowledge of anatomy to reason and improvise. This counter-principle follows from the belief that a surgeon must be self-confident and have a "big ego" and demonstrate that he can handle anything.

In reality, situations of emergency requiring improvisation in unexpected circumstances are very rare: most good surgeons generally know exactly what they are getting into before the patient is in the operating room. And in the case of elective (non-emergency) procedures (as in the case being described here) there is knowledge of the medical situation well in advance of having to do something about it. The chances for success or survival in a surgical procedure are naturally much higher when the patient is in the hands of a surgeon experienced in such procedures, and that is why a surgeon is under informal pressure not to take on something he knows little about.

On the other hand, highly specialized surgeons (such as cardiac surgeons) admit to getting bored now and then with doing the same procedures over and over again, and they are tempted by the rare opportunities to try their hand at something new. As one of the other surgeons speculated, perhaps that is why Dr. Bush was so insistent about operating on the little girl. Moreover, he had lately been encountering a great deal of resistance from the hospital staff, who complained that he was not around Lakeside often or long enough to take care of his cardiac surgery patients. Since it was hard to get enough cardiac surgery referrals to keep him going at Lakeside alone (most of the medical doctors referred their patients who needed heart surgery to one of the larger medical centers), he had been forced to spread out his surgical practice in several different hospitals across a wide geographical area. In fact, he occupied a major training and administrative position at one of the other hospitals, which meant that he was frequently away from Lakeside and left much of the postoperative care of his patients to the judgment of his residents and interns, a situation that caused concern among many of the staff members at Lakeside. Some had observed the mortality and morbidity rates of his cardiac surgery practice to be uncomfortably high, and so, they explained, they were especially upset with his absence and unavailability at the hospital. Some of his colleagues speculated that Bush had become annoyed with the criticism that was directed toward him, and lately he seemed to pay little attention to their complaints.

The little girl scheduled for surgery was not in any immediate distress, in fact she was an athletic child, but her family physician had decided that it was a good time to repair the heart defect, which would eventually interfere with the child's activities. It is not known why he referred the child to Bush rather than to Children's Hospital.

Bush had arranged for a special pediatric anesthesiologist from Children's Hospital to come over to Lakeside for the case, since none of their own anesthesiologists had ever done any open heart cases on children. The visiting anesthesiologist, Dr. Dentler, had his own doubts about doing the case at Lakeside. He had met the child's parents the night before surgery when he had stopped in the girl's room to do the customary preoperative exam, and as he later admitted, he had been tempted to say, "Hey, why don't you move your daughter over to Children's Hospital." But Dentler later explained that saying such a thing was entirely out of the question: making a remark like that would have cost him dearly in his professional career.

As Dentler later described, his anxiety soared as they began the operation. He had wanted to insert an atrial line at the start of the surgery, and Bush had autocratically refused. Dentler was worried: he didn't see how they could proceed safely with the operation without the line, but he feared that if he threatened to withdraw from the case unless the line was inserted, it would turn into a "battle of egos," and Bush had a great deal more power than he. So, as Dentler later told the story, he had let Bush save face by saying, "Sir, I know that you're probably right, but I would feel very uncomfortable if we don't put in the atrial line to be extra safe." Bush had agreed, then, but once they got into the heart the anesthesiologist once again saw cause for alarm.

They had expected to find only an atrial-septal defect, which is a common problem and easy to repair, but once the heart was exposed they could see that this little girl also had an additional cardiac abnormality in the configuration of the pulmonary veins leading from her heart. It looked as if she had an unusual version of another fairly common abnormality known as partial anomalous pulmonary venous return, but her vessels did not exactly follow the classic arrangement of the abnormality, and the situation was not entirely clear. Furthermore, because Bush had originally anticipated only an atrial-septal defect, he had approached the heart through an incision that did not lend itself well either to observing or repairing the pulmonary veins.

Dentler felt immediately that they should just close up and refer the little girl to an expert at Children's Hospital. The child had been doing very well until now, and was in no immediate need of surgery. The operation she needed could best be done by one of the pediatric cardiac surgeons who had experience with this sort of thing. But as Dentler later explained, he could see that Bush was not about to give up that easily, and so what could he do? It was not within his power as an anesthesiologist to argue with the surgeon. He could (and indeed had) argue about the insertion of the atrial line, since that was a matter of anesthesia. But a judgment about surgery could only come from the surgeon, he felt, and Bush would have to decide if he could in good conscience do the operation, and the burden of the outcome would have to rest on his (the surgeon's) shoulders. Dentler admitted to feeling terrible: he knew that if they attempted surgery and it turned out badly he would feel regret at his participation in the case, but he kept telling himself that it was not his responsibility to interfere with the surgeon's decision, and he would have to mind his own business.

Word of the surprise finding had now reached Anna Stewart, the cardiology fellow who had done the original diagnostic tests, and she was summoned down to the operating room and asked to bring some books and charts about the abnormality with instructions about surgical approaches to the repair. Bush had already figured out a surgical strategy, and he explained that he just wanted to look at a few diagrams to check out his ideas. Dr. Stewart changed quickly into a surgical suit and brought the books into the operating room. She was visibly upset. She felt partly to blame for this disaster, because she had not predicted this situation in her pre-operative diagnosis. Still, it was always hard to know exactly what one would find in these situations until the heart was actually exposed, which is why she agreed with the others that this kind of operation was best done at a hospital specializing in these procedures. When she joined the others in the operating room, she was not at all sure about what was going on in the child's heart and circulatory system, and she felt that Bush did not know enough to operate. But, as she told one of the interns standing nearby, she could hardly try to dissuade Bush. For one thing, it could be argued that *she* had made the first mistake in the misdiagnosis, and since she was only just beginning her cardiology training, she could hardly tell the surgeon how to run his own practice. If the Chief of Cardiology had been around, she felt that she might have been able to get him to intervene, but he was out of town at a medical conference.

As Bush had explained in the operating room, there were three choices open to them. They could stop the surgery and close the chest and send the child to Children's Hospital. Anna Stewart and Dentler indicated through their looks to one another that this was what they preferred. The second option was to try to reach one of the several pediatric cardiac surgeons in the city by telephone, and either get one of them to come to the hospital right away, or get their advice over the telephone about how to complete the operation. Stewart indicated to her intern friend that this was her second choice of actions. Or, Bush concluded, they could just use their heads and improvise, and Bush was sure he knew what to do. It was obvious that all of the surgeons in the room (Bush's first assistant and the two residents) were in agreement—they were ready to go ahead with the surgery. After all, they laughed, a smart bunch of fellows like themselves should be able to handle the problem. As they resumed the procedure Dr. Stewart left the operating room, telling the intern that she was frightened at what might happen, and hoping to find a way to intervene. She could think of only two staff doctors who might be persuaded and in a position to do something: one was Dr. Cameron, the Chief of Anesthesiology, and the other was the one cardiac surgeon on the hospital staff whom she considered approachable in such matters.

She admitted to the intern that she was afraid of Cameron. She knew that he objected to the entire cardiac service as it was presently constituted at Lakeside, and that he wished it would be reorganized or terminated. And even though she was not a surgeon herself, as a cardiologist she had to work with the surgeons and she depended on the cardiac surgery service to be able to do the diagnostic procedures she was learning about. So she felt that Cameron was likely to associate her with the larger cardiac group that he opposed.

She found him talking to someone in the OR corridor, and nervously approached him. He snapped at her when she raised the issue, for he was already informed and obviously upset about it. He had heard about what was going on in the thoracic operating room from the visiting anesthesiologist, and although he didn't approve of what they were doing he was not going to get involved in an argument now. "You had no business doing that operation. What do you know about pediatric surgery? A child isn't a small adult. You can't treat a child like a miniature adult. I'll tell you, Dr. Stewart, if *I* were the surgeon in charge of the case, I would swallow my pride and admit that I was out of my depth and close up. But Bush's ego is too fragile—he's not going to listen to me anyway, so what's the use of my getting into an argument with him now? While he's operating?" He walked away, and the cardiologist was left alone standing in the corridor.

The only option left was to try to reach Dr. Tolman, the cardiac surgeon she liked. She paged him and when he came to the telephone she explained the situation and asked if he couldn't step into the OR, look over Bush's shoulder and, as one cardiac surgeon to another, suggest that they get help.

The surgeon sympathized but explained that there was no way he could do that. Whatever he might personally think of Bush, and he didn't particularly like what Bush was doing in this case, he still had to work with the man, and he couldn't go sticking his nose into Bush's operations. Anyway, a surgeon's "ego," he explained, had to be protected, and you couldn't just tell someone with a knife in his hand that he should stop the case.

To their relief and surprise, Dentler and Stewart watched the operation go smoothly, and the child was returned to the Intensive Care Unit doing fairly well. Whatever would happen in the long run, at least the child had made it through the operation. The two young doctors knew that they were going to pay for their doubts, so they voiced a steady stream of compliments and congratulations to Bush for his good judgment and skill.

Now it was the surgeon's chance to turn on the cardiologist. When the group reconvened that afternoon for their weekly cardiac conference, one of Bush's residents questioned Anna Stewart: "How come you didn't catch the abnormality in your examination and diagnostic tests?"

Stewart had no answer, and she kept thanking Bush and the other surgeons for "bailing us out of our mistake." As she later explained, she felt that it had been an honest mistake for a cardiologist to make, and that the surgeons were the ones at fault for insisting on completing the operation; still, she knew that she would have to take a beating for showing doubt in the operating room. In a barely controlled mood of triumph, Bush cracked his chewing gum and interrupted the surgical resident who was criticizing Anna Stewart: "Well, after all, let's drop it. It was just the little girl who counted."

Doctors who work together in a teaching hospital are always in a position to observe their colleagues' performances. Even across status and specialty lines, the activities of each doctor can be viewed by the others. Anesthesiologists can watch the work of surgeons; medical residents and attending doctors suspiciously eye one another; and cardiologists and surgeons negotiate decisions about heart surgery. Furthermore, the house officers and teaching staff produce a hospital-wide network of gossip and information about all of the doctors and their cases.

Not only are doctors continuously put in a position of witnessing each other's practices, but they are also frequently required to collaborate or participate in activities initiated by other doctors, whether or not they approve of these procedures. Anesthesiologists and residents are expected to serve and assist the staff surgeons whose cases they are assigned to; attending phyicians are expected to trust and allow the residents some freedom to do what they wish with patients, and cardiologists are frequently asked to cooperate in the diagnostic and postoperative treatment of patients whose surgical procedures they personally oppose.

Under such circumstances, it might be expected that doctors would be exposed to frequent moral dilemmas about collaborating in activities about which they have doubts. For though a doctor may personally doubt the wisdom of a particular procedure, physicians who refuse to collaborate with their colleagues often find themselves working at a professional and financial disadvantage. The freedom and ability to do their own work easily and profitably usually depends upon the good feelings and relationships which doctors enjoy with their colleagues.

The doctor's potential moral uneasiness is relieved by the professional etiquette and ideology which helps him through such moments. For doctors are provided with a wide range of collective rationales for not interrupting, and even agreeing to participate in, dubious procedures and decisions.

The incident described above illustrates how doctors may use their different specializations and lower statuses to justify their cooperation in a procedure to which they object. The general principle in medicine is that each doctor should attend to his own store and treat his colleagues like honorable gentlemen, as individuals who can be trusted to act competently and decently. And, if a superior orders a procedure with an unfortunate outcome, the subordinates cannot be blamed for carrying out orders.

The medical etiquette that guides doctors into avoiding

passing judgment or intervening in a colleague's work is supported by a further kind of professional justification. Doctors often argue that practicing medicine or surgery is like practicing an art rather than a science. Such an argument is useful to doctors in an uncomfortable situation, for if sound medical and surgical judgments (coming out of an "artistic" process) are to rest on clinical judgment and a physician's personal intuition about each patient and case, then clearly no doctor can be held accountable for not following a generally agreed-upon standard of action for each sort of case.

As one training staff member voiced the common expression: "There is no right and wrong in medicine. There are several ways of doing things. Different ways work better in different situations. Medicine is not exactly a science, and each doctor must be given the freedom to use the method which in his own experience works best." On the occasion of this remark, the doctor was defending his medical residents for failing to carry out the standard treatment for an Emergency Room patient in pulmonary edema. The residents had gotten into an argument with the attending doctor about the cause of the edema, and had failed to treat the life-threatening symptoms in accordance with the usual practice in such situations. One can imagine the implications of such a belief: if medicine is an "art" and if there is no right and wrong in medicine, then clearly no one can be held accountable for mistakes.

The argument about medicine being an "art" is invoked by doctors only in an ad hoc fashion, and when it is convenient. For, on other occasions, statistical evidence or scientific findings will also be cited by doctors to justify activities. For example, in order to defend retrospectively a procedure that turned out badly in a particular instance (for example, a death in surgery) many doctors often move the argument into discussions about "probabilities" which made the surgery the right choice (despite the outcome), and on these occasions their arguments assume that medicine operates on a scientific model.

Chiefs of hospital services and department heads have their

own distinctive sets of justifications for not intervening in poor medical practice. These individuals are in a good position to know about the mistakes and incompetence of their staff members, for their residents and interns report to them each day about difficulties in hospital cases.

Under these circumstances, one might guess that a department head would often be faced with the responsibility for removing or censuring a doctor on his staff. But such incidents happen extremely rarely. Only once every several years at Lakeside did the hospital even consider revoking the admitting or operating privileges of any attending doctor for reasons of incompetence. Doctors who were openly acknowledged by the chiefs to be dangerous or incompetent were instead allowed to remain on the staff, and various justifications were cited. The most common explanation offered by the chiefs at Lakeside was that if they were to suspend a doctor's hospital privileges, the doctor would do even more harm. The reasoning went like this: when a bad doctor admitted his patients to Lakeside, there were residents and staff around making sure that the patient was treated correctly. Similarly, it was argued that the chief resident of the surgical service made sure that the most experienced residents were assigned to assist in the operations of the worst surgeons, in order to rescue the situation.

On the other hand, went this familiar argument, if the hospital privileges of the incompetent doctors were suspended, these doctors would either do their poor work without correction in their own offices, or else they would admit their patients to a worse hospital where there would be no residents or staff to look over their shoulders. And so, concluded the Chief of Medicine, the patients were best protected by making sure that incompetent doctors were *kept* on the staff. Interestingly enough, the question of getting an incompetent doctor's general license to practice revoked (so that he could not move his incompetent work into his office or another hospital) was never seen to be a possible alternative. Such an action is simply not taken in the world of medicine. Most doctors think of regulation in terms of keeping their own backyards in order. Their backyards may extend, on occasion, to include their hospital, but most do not feel the obligation ever to meddle beyond.

They rarely resort to such drastic measures as suspending licenses and privileges. Indeed, the hospital department heads argued that they had to handle their staff members with kid gloves, and had to be very spare in offering criticism or advice. The explanation advanced here was that unless they were very gentle with the less capable private doctors affiliated with their departments, these doctors wouldn't come to them for help when they were in trouble. For example, the Chief of Surgery at Lakeside explained that he couldn't be very openly critical of the doctors on his staff because he wanted them to feel comfortable enough to call him in on the disasters. He told the following story to illustrate his point:

"Last year one of our elderly surgeons was doing a sigmoidoscopy [an examination of the colon and large intestine with the use of an optical instrument inserted via the rectum] on a spinster-teacher and he accidentally perforated her colon, and her peritoneal cavity got filled up with feces. He was a wreck. He didn't know what to do and he called me up and said he needed help. The woman had cancer and was going to need a colostomy anyway, but now she needed to have emergency surgery.

"So I met him out in the hall and I said, 'Relax, have a cup of coffee, let me handle the whole thing.' So we went in and I did all the talking. I said 'You have a cancer. You will need surgery and will have to use an ostomy bag. This should be done as soon as possible in any case. In the course of your examination a technical problem happened and a hole was made in your colon, so it is now necessary for us to proceed immediately.'

"She agreed. The elderly surgeon and I took her to the OR together and I started the surgery. He was assisting me but halfway through he said, 'I have to leave the room, I'm a nervous wreck.' So I told him, 'Sit down, have a cup of coffee, relax.' He went into the lounge for a cup of coffee and I did the operation by myself. He collected the fee and the patient never knew that I had anything to do with it. So that is why I can't be too hard on these surgeons."

Certain doctors, by virtue of their special positions in the hospital, are likely to know about others doctors' "disasters." Patients who have been poorly treated with serious consequence will eventually come under the care of the Chief Cardiologist in the Coronary Care Unit or the Chief of Infectious Diseases. Like the hospital pathologists who do the autopsies, these doctors are the ultimate recipients of other doctors' mistakes. Like the chiefs of medicine and surgery, they too argue that they must be gentle with their criticisms of other doctors, or else they will not be consulted when they are badly needed.

For example, the Chief of Infectious Diseases at Lakeside explained that he had to be tactful when dealing with careless surgeons whose patients developed surgical wound infections. "When the postoperative patient develops an infection —even when I'm sure that it's a wound infection which is the surgeon's fault—I can't come right out and say that to the surgeon. I have to say, 'Well, it's possible that it *could* be a wound infection.' You know you have to be very diplomatic to do this job at all."

Still another service chief echoed the refrain that criticism or the pointing out of mistakes could not be done directly. He argued: "You can't say things to people directly. They won't listen to you. It's all indirect. You have to plant people in strategic places to suggest things to bad doctors. Once a doctor gets his license to operate, no one's going to stop him from doing anything. It's easier to practice medicine than to keep a driver's license. And so-called peer review is a big farce. When we review cases in the Utilization Review Committee we don't even bother to look at the case records of the worst doctors—we already know that they'll be terrible. And what would be the use of calling them up before the committee? They're not going to change anyway, so why waste the time? And if we go through the cases of the good doctors, what is there to gain? Chances are, if the reasonably good doctors have made a mistake they're already aware of it, even before we go through their records. So what's the point of the review?"

Despite the fact that doctors are trusted by the public to "police" themselves, in situation after situation we may observe justifications, explanations, rationalizations and excuses for not intervening in what is seen as other doctors' medical incompetence. Even the formal mechanisms of peer control are rarely and ineffectively used. Mortality Review Meetings actually provide comfort and excuses for doctors' errors; the worst mistakes are ignored, and blame is shifted to the patient. The Utilization Review Committee doesn't bother to examine the charts of the worst doctors, and sees no point in reviewing those of the responsible physicians. Those at the *bottom* of the hierarchy plead inability to speak out and challenge the orders of their superiors. Those at the *top* of the hierarchy argue that they must be diplomatic, in order to maintain any control at all. Members of specialties plead inability to speak out on the activities of doctors in another field. Members of the same specialty explain that they must mind their own business to be able to work with their colleagues. Bad doctors are kept on the staff so that they will be kept out of worse trouble, and finally, it is argued that medicine or surgery is an "art," with no rights and wrongs, and each doctor must be left to act on the basis of his hunches and personal experience.

These justifications often sound convincing, and are sincerely meant, but doctors are unable to regulate the quality of medical care. They are unlikely to censure those of their profession who are incompetent; and they are unlikely to assess and identify medical mistakes. In addition to all of the explanations and justifications described earlier, those doctors who are frankest will also admit that the structure of financial rewards works against physicians' criticizing one another for bad practices. The words of one cardiologist are illuminating:

"I'm opposed to doing coronary bypass surgery except in cases of intractable pain. The keynote address at the American College of Cardiology meetings this year confirmed my feeling. Believe me, I look for a good reason to do that kind of surgery even when the patient is not in intractable pain because it would increase my business fourfold. But I honestly can't come up with any reason for it.

"So when the surgeons ask me to do a catheterization in a case that I don't think should go to surgery, and I say, 'No, I don't think surgery is justified in this instance,' then they're going to take their business elsewhere, and have someone else do it. And then they're not going to invite me to consult or do a catheterization even in the cases that I think call for surgery. If I won't do it whenever they want, they'll find someone else. They figure, if he doesn't like doing the procedure, don't give him *any* to do.

"And in those cardiac conferences Dalton presents his private cases which we haven't even had a chance to examine. How can we argue with him when he didn't give us a chance to look at the patient? It's a fait accompli. So I try to save my arguments for patients where it might do some good— when I can have a chance to examine the patient and say something based on hard evidence.

"Let me give you an example of how this works. There's a fellow who just died up in the Intensive Care Unit this morning who shouldn't have had heart surgery when he did. He had an infection and was spiking fever and the surgery should have been postponed. He probably had endocarditis [an infection of the heart tissue] at the time of surgery, and it should have been postponed, but the surgeon needed to do a case this week in order to keep up the minimum case load required to maintain the thoracic service.

"I couldn't say anything about the case. I did the catheterization on the patient, but he developed the infection afterwards, and at that time I was no longer involved in the case. I'm not invited to consult on these cases after the catheterization, and there's no pay for it. The rule is that only a certain number of consultants can get paid. I get paid as a consultant only to do the catheterization before surgery and then they hire Dr. Howell as the consulting cardiologist for postoperative care because he's their friend and he's old and doesn't come to the hospital often and won't interfere with the way they want to run the cases. I can't stick my nose in it because it's not my patient any more. The case belongs to the surgeons and I have no right to interfere, nor do I get paid for it.

"But I will tell you this. If I hadn't been up in the Intensive Care Unit this morning and noticed that patient's tachycardia and arrhythmias they wouldn't have even known that he was dying."

6

KEEPING THE PATIENT UNINFORMED AND CLOSING THE RANKS

. . . The stature of a physician in the eyes of his patient is a significant factor in the patient's response to illness and in his willingness to accept a recommendation for a potentially uncomfortable or dangerous procedure. Should the resident or intern disagree with an attending physician's assessment of a problem or suggestion of therapy, this should not be discussed within the patient's hearing. Likewise, the patient's confidence in the physician should not be undermined by innuendo or actual disparagement of the physician's judgment. It is essential to avoid caustic or intemperate comments in the chart, which is today almost a public document . . .

*—From a memorandum issued to interns
and residents in* _____ *Hospital.*

One of the basic rules in medical practice is that patients should not be informed of disagreement among doctors concerning their diagnosis and treatment. Even when medical consultants or house officers do not agree with the decisions of the attending doctor, they are expressly forbidden to communicate their doubts to the patient. Asked why differences of opinion are kept hidden from patients, most doctors will argue that patients would be upset were they to know about disagreement about their treatment. Doctors generally agree that all the physicians working on a case should "maintain a party line" to feed to the patient in consideration of his feelings. However sincere they may be in wanting to spare the patient from worry, it is also clear that doctors serve their own interests when they withhold information from the patient. Indeed, protecting themselves from the discomfort and inconvenience of sharing all the information with the patient frequently takes precedence over protecting the patient's emotional or even physical well-being.

There are two kinds of information that doctors routinely withhold from patients: one kind has to do with facts about the patient's illness; the other kind has to do with evaluations of the competence or performance of the other doctors involved in the case, or the wisdom of the treatment that other doctors have recommended. Although doctors rationalize withholding such information (of both sorts) on the grounds of "protecting" the patient from upsetting information, in fact they are more precisely protecting themselves and their colleagues. For the less that patients know about the problems of their treatment and the faults or errors of their doctors, the less able they are to disagree or make trouble for their physicians.

Keeping the patient uninformed and closing ranks with regard to information are two of the ways that doctors limit the power and autonomy of patients. Despite rationalizations, this is often done by doctors to help one another rather than to help the patient.

Many doctors, for example, argue that certain kinds of information (such as disagreement over diagnosis) must be kept hidden from the patient because the patient wishes and needs to view his or her physician as infallible. But such a justification for hiding dissenting opinions often warrants skepticism. One surgeon, for example, suspected that an elderly patient had pancreatic cancer, and he told her that an exploratory operation should be performed immediately, the next day if possible. Following this announcement the patient became extremely upset and the surgeon arranged for a psychiatric consultation. After his interview with the patient, the psychiatrist urged the surgeon to postpone the operation for a week. He believed that the patient's symptoms might disappear or be otherwise explained and that if the patient did indeed have pancreatic cancer, knowing it a week later would not change her prognosis. By postponing the operation they might spare her from a dreaded experience. The surgeon agreed with the psychiatrist's reasoning, but refused to delay the surgery. He maintained that the patient needed to have complete confidence in him, and that if he were to change the plan it might jeopardize her faith in him. The surgical exploration turned out to reveal nothing but a benign mass that would have disappeared by itself.

In keeping information secret and hidden from the patient, doctors are occasionally more concerned with saving their own faces than with the patient's feelings. The following incident, described in some detail, illustrates such a situation.

A thirty-five-year-old female patient, who was a biochemist by occupation, was told over several years by many doctors that her recurrent abdominal pains were merely "functional" (psychological) and that diagnostic x-rays were unnecessary. Even when she appeared on several consecutive nights in the Emergency Room complaining of severe pain she was given a mild tranquilizer and sent home. But when she arrived the following week in her doctor's office, obviously jaundiced, her complaints could no longer be passed off as the fabrications of what the doctor imagined to be a hysterical woman. Nervously, her doctor insisted that she be admitted to the hospital on the spot, insisting that "the buck stops here" (despite the fact that *he* had been the one who had discounted the symptoms all along). Diagnostic x-rays were done to see whether she had gastrointestinal or gall bladder disease. During the gall bladder x-ray, her liver failed to release the visualizing dye as it normally should have, and so it was evident that there was something wrong with her hepato-biliary system. A simple explanation might have been that her liver was temporarily misfunctioning only because of gall bladder disease and an obstructive stone in her bile duct. But because of results which appeared in laboratory studies of her blood, the doctor suspected that she had an intrinsic liver disease, independent of any disorder of the gall bladder. He informed her that a liver biopsy should be done immediately. When she questioned him about the procedure he admitted that it carried a very small risk of serious hemorrhaging, but boasted that she need not worry—he had done hundreds and never lost a single patient.

Since her illness had gone unattended for so long, the patient saw no reason to rush into a liver biopsy. She proposed, instead, that a specialist in liver diseases be consulted before proceeding with the test, and she also asked whether they might delay the biopsy for a few days to see if her liver function tests would return to normal, for such a change would indicate that her liver malfunction was merely temporary and secondary to gall bladder disease. If they could wait a few days, a liver biopsy might therefore be avoided.

Her doctor responded to these suggestions by informing her that *he* was the doctor and *she* the patient, and that he was practically certain that she suffered from chronic active hepatitis, a very serious disease, and that she had better not delay the procedure since only a liver biopsy could confirm the diagnosis. Furthermore, if he were correct, she would have to be put on a regimen of steroids.

Yielding to the pressure and having checked around town to make sure that the doctor was well regarded, the patient agreed to the procedure. The biopsy was performed with the customary joking of her physician. She was awake during the procedure; a paper towel was placed over her eyes so she couldn't watch, and the physician inserted a needle into her liver, in order to withdraw a sample of the organ. Since she experienced no pain in the procedure the doctor tried to humor her out of her annoyance with him by complimenting her. As he placed the specimen in a jar he joked that they had done so well he could take her around the country to demonstrate tolerance for liver biopsies. She replied that she had better things to do with her time.

After being returned to her room, the patient was visited by two other patients on the floor under the care of the same doctor who were scheduled to have *their* livers biopsied the next day. They had come by to find out what the test was really like, and one remarked: "There's something strange about this. All you hear on this floor is liver biopsy, liver biopsy. All of his patients can't have the same disease." The patient shared the others' suspicion when she learned of the doctor's widespread use of the test, and she wondered whether he was especially interested in discovering diseases of the liver.

The night after the procedure, the patient was unable to reach her doctor to hear the results of the test but she managed to persuade an intern assigned to her case (he had just moved to the city and was lonely and she promised to find him some friends) to bring her his medical books so that she could read about the varieties of hepatitis. Looking up chronic active hepatitis, she was stunned to read that the disease had no cure and that it was usually fatal within a few years. When the intern came to collect his books she pointed to the section she had read and asked when she would know the results of the liver biopsy. The intern looked distressed and explained that he had not realized the seriousness of the disease or he would not have let her read about the illness unprepared for the news. But he urged her not to jump to conclusions and asked her not to say anything about it, or he might get into trouble for having shown her his books. As for the results of the biopsy, he told her that he was not allowed as an intern to relay that information to her, and she would have to wait until her own doctor discussed it with her.

The next day was the start of the July fourth holiday weekend and the patient was told that her doctor could not be reached and would be unavailable for a couple of days. Over the holiday the patient tried to find out the results of the test, indicating that she knew the seriousness of the suspected disease. But the house officers and the associate covering for her physician all apologized and explained that she would have to wait until her own doctor returned. She expressed fright and concern about their evasiveness, but was unable to obtain any further information. During the two-day wait she became increasingly depressed about their reluctance to tell her the results of the test. When her doctor finally returned he was vague about the test results, and claimed that he had not yet had a chance to examine the specimen himself, and had only heard a report over the telephone.

Upon looking at her newest blood tests, however, he expressed puzzlement and discomfort, and quietly remarked, "this is certainly a surprise." With seeming embarrassment rather than obvious pleasure he informed the patient that her liver function as measured by her most recent blood tests had now returned to normal, and this indicated that after all (as she had suggested in requesting the delay of the biopsy) her jaundice and liver disorder had only been a temporary problem caused by a stone in the bile duct. She could now be scheduled for surgery the following day. Asked if she had any preference for surgeons, she replied, with obvious mixed relief and annoyance, "A competent one—it's about time this case was handled properly." He joked back: "Oh, I thought I'd get you a surgeon who needs the money."

Even after the doctor seemed to change his mind about the illness the patient was still concerned about the mysterious results of the liver biopsy. When her doctor had suspected liver disease only a few days before, he had told her that with such a condition she would be unable to tolerate surgery. Because of all that had happened she had little confidence that the matter had been adequately resolved, and she was reluctant to agree to an operation until she was certain of what the biopsy showed. Since she was to have surgery the next day, she had extracted a promise from her doctor that he would call her and tell her the test results that evening, as soon as he had a chance to examine the specimen. But he assured her that there was no need for her to worry—he was certain that her liver was fine. When the doctor failed to call that evening she tried to reach his answering service every half hour, but was repeatedly told that he was unavailable. Seeing no alternative, and aware of the carelessness that had characterized her treatment thus far, the patient refused to sign the consent form or take the preoperative sleeping medication until she heard the results of the test. At midnight, when she refused to go to bed and threatened to make a scene in the hospital corridor unless her doctor became available, a furious resident finally placed the call and was immediately connected with the physician. Still, her doctor was reluctant to elaborate and all he would say was, "Don't worry, the biopsy didn't show anything wrong with your liver."

After the operation the patient continued to be puzzled about why all the doctors had been so evasive about reporting the test results, when doing so would seemingly have assured her that she had a curable rather than an incurable disease and would have saved her from two days of extreme distress. As the time came to be released from the hospital she asked her physician if she could read her chart, but even after obtaining his permission (he boasted that he had nothing to hide—he had never been sued), when she went to the nurses' station and reached out to take the record, a nurse stopped her hand and pushed it away. Obviously annoyed with the patient's assertiveness, the nurse smugly informed her that even though her medical physician had agreed, when her surgeon had been informed of her request to see the chart he had left word that she was not to be allowed to look at it.

She returned to her room, furious and even more determined to see the chart. She knew that it was ultimately within her legal rights to obtain a copy, and it was just a question of how much trouble and expense they would put her through. She was curious to see whether the surgeon, who was making his morning rounds, would mention that he had blocked her access to the chart, and she decided not to raise the matter at first but to await his response. He came by moments later, and after silently checking on her wound, he turned to go, having made no reference to his veto of her request. She called to him as he was stepping out the door:

"Dr. Williams—I understand you object to my seeing my chart. Would you mind telling me why?"

He looked unperturbed and replied, "It's not that I object. But it's not our policy to show our patients their charts. And our patients don't want to see their charts."

She raised her eyebrows in mock surprise and answered sweetly, "But *I* want to see my chart. That's why I asked to see it."

A smile of contempt crossed his face. "Why do you want to see your chart? It's really not very interesting reading."

She replied: "Because I'd like to know all the facts pertinent to my illness."

He began to show signs of impatience and the placid smile looked more like a sneer. "Well, I'm sorry, but it's not a good idea and it wouldn't mean anything to you anyway. You wouldn't understand anything you were reading and then you'd have a million questions."

He had started to leave, but she felt that she now had an advantage. "Don't worry, Dr. Williams. If I have any questions I promise I won't ask *you* for any answers."

Assuming his usual look of icy imperturbability, he turned to go. "Go ahead, read your chart. I don't care."

The patient waited triumphantly in her room for fifteen minutes, thinking that even terrible experiences could have their better moments, and then she marched out to the nurses' station. She thought it would be more effective to say nothing as she helped herself to her record, but she happily took in the sight of the glaring nurses who silently watched her. A resident standing nearby remarked: "You know, even when *doctors* are patients they don't see their own charts."

She answered cheerfully, feeling that she could afford to be generous now. "That's their problem, not mine."

After returning to her room she shut the door behind her and climbed into bed with the chart. (She always kept the door closed for privacy and had insisted that the doctors and nurses knock before entering her room; they had complied but it irritated them.) Hurriedly, she searched through the record for the report on the liver biopsy. She discovered that it was only a single line written on an otherwise blank sheet of paper. It merely read: "No analysis, Specimen Insufficient For Diagnosis."

The evasiveness of the doctors was finally explained to the patient. No one had wanted her to learn that the procedure had been a total waste. The physician, through miscalculation or bad luck, had failed to insert the needle into the proper place and had therefore missed getting a proper sample. Rather than let her know that her doctor had failed to complete the procedure successfully, the house officers and covering physician had instead allowed her to believe for two days that she was dying. And when directly asked about the test results, her own doctor had evasively lied by saying, "The test didn't show anything wrong with your liver," since the test had shown nothing at all.

Such a bending of the truth, or the use of misleading remarks, is common in the reports that doctors give to patients. As one chief of surgery explained, when a surgeon performs an appendectomy on a patient who turns out to have a normal appendix, rather than admit the situation to the family, he may very well say, with misleading accuracy, "That appendix was red, all right." And when a patient dies in cardiac surgery partly because of the clumsiness of the surgeons, the family is likely instead to be told: "We did our best but her heart was so weak and far gone that she just couldn't make it through the operation."

With increasing concern about malpractice suits and rising insurance costs, doctors have become even more cautious about sharing information with their patients. New patient consent forms and requirements are actually more specifically designed to protect physicians against liability than to make sure that patients are well informed about the procedures they submit to. And even though the medical chart is the primary source of information used in the patient's treatment, and the main channel of communication between staff members collaborating on a case (who may never talk directly but merely write notes to each other), doctors are becoming more and more reluctant to record certain kinds of information in medical charts lest the record be used against them in some future lawsuit.

As patients demand more information and access to their medical records, the chart is more frequently constructed as a "case record" having more to do with protecting the doctor from lawsuit than anything else.

As doctors increasingly feel abused, persecuted, insufficiently appreciated, and misunderstood by their patients and the public, they are closing ranks more tightly than ever. As one department chief explained: "I don't believe patients should be told when they've acquired an iatrogenic [physician-produced] illness. They just can't understand the risks of the procedures we do, so why should we tell them when they've become sick from something we've tried? So they can sue us?"

At the same time that doctors draw together to protect each other, their concern with medical standards is becoming shaped less by a determination to avoid mistakes than by a desire to avoid lawsuits. As one intern explained to another in the Lakeside Hospital Emergency Room: "Every time a patient comes in here complaining of a headache, I make him lie down and I do a lumbar [spinal] puncture. If they want to come in here and bother us with their headaches, let them have their spinal cords punctured and let them lie here without moving for a few hours. I'm not gonna let anyone walk out of here with an undiagnosed subarachnoid bleed so they can sue me later. If they have a headache, just give them the works—l.p. [do a lumbar puncture] them all—we're here to protect ourselves, no one else."

Although rising fears of lawsuits have made doctors more cautious about sharing information with patients, the fear of being sued has made at least some doctors more likely to argue with one another about questionable procedures for which they are personally liable. As one anesthesiologist explained: "We never used to argue with surgeons. Whatever they wanted to do was okay with us. But now that we're getting included in the lawsuits over malpractice in surgery, we're starting to fight with them about what they're doing. Now that I know I can be sued, I'm not going to let some surgeon do whatever he pleases, and I'm not going to do whatever they tell me. I tell the surgeon he can do it my way or he can just do the whole thing himself."

On one occasion the department of surgery at Lakeside Hospital devoted a session of Surgical Grand Rounds (a weekly hospital conference for the continuing education of staff surgeons) to the issue of lawsuits. A lawyer had been invited to lecture the staff on how to avoid lawsuits. Not surprisingly, the lawyer's advice had nothing at all to do with how to avoid mistakes but rather how to avoid being sued.

The guest speaker was the legal adviser to a nearby medical center, and seemed to enjoy the opportunity to tell doctors what to do. Over and over again he repeated one point: "Your patients won't sue you, no matter what you do to them, as long as they love you. They'll only sue you if they hate you. Be courteous, have a little humility and they won't sue you. And what really sets a patient off against a doctor he hates is a big bill. When a patient is deciding whether or not to sue a doctor, it's the big bill which is often the straw that breaks the camel's back. So if you have a patient who hasn't paid a bill, and you know he's mad at you for something, by all means, *drop the bill!*

"Some doctors think that dropping a bill is an admission of guilt. But it's not. In fact you'll look much better in court if you can say, 'I dropped the bill because I knew that Mr. So-and-So was not satisfied with his treatment, and I didn't think that he should have to pay for something he's not happy with.' "

The lawyer next discussed the problem of charts, and how doctors made themselves more or less vulnerable to lawsuits by how they kept medical records.

"Many doctors try to change what they've written in a chart, or leave things out, or use abbreviations like DNR for Do Not Resuscitate, because they're afraid the charts will be used as incriminating evidence against them. But if you do this and you get called up for something seven years from now, you'll be your own fool's witness because you won't remember what the hell happened in the case."

After questions were invited from the audience, one surgeon seemed to create discomfort among the group by describing with obvious distress how one of his patients was threatening to sue him. After relating the circumstances of the case while the other surgeons looked impatiently up at the ceiling or down at their shoes (for this doctor was truly an embarrassment to the staff and always in trouble; and besides, he wore garish clothing and yellow suits) he wanted the lawyer to tell him whether he could be found guilty of malpractice. The Chief of Surgery interrupted the discussion and suggested that he continue the conversation later over coffee.

The lawyer concluded his lecture by reminding the surgeons that at his medical center there were very few lawsuits: "Only three during all of last year. And why? Because of the mystique of our hospital. Patients think that doctors can do no wrong at our hospital, even if they go home crippled. So just remember, if they love you they won't sue you and if they hate you, they will. It's all a matter of public relations."

In considering the legal and monetary considerations that encourage doctors to withhold information from patients, still another motivating element must not be overlooked: this is physician control of the situation. Because they are accustomed to complete autonomy in their work, doctors typically become highly uncomfortable in situations that are beyond their control. In these instances they frequently attempt to reassert control in some self-consoling way, even if such efforts do not best serve the interests of their patients. In the next account a physician explains why he withholds information from patients when he is unable to cure them. The explanations of this physician are illuminating because they tell us about the attitudes some doctors have toward patients and about the ways physicians may rationalize their behavior. When asked why they hide information from patients, doctors typically cite the same proverbial situation: the case of the patient who is dying from cancer, passing over all the other kinds of cases in which information is withheld for convenience, control, or self-protection.

By assuming the right and privilege to withhold information and to interpret the psychological needs of the patient, the physician may be motivated by a desire to solve his own wounded sense of power and competency in a medical case he could not successfully control. But in treating his own damaged pride, the physician fails to consider how his tactics seriously harm the patient. For by not admitting to the patient that he cannot help him and that he is dying, the physician deprives the patient of the opportunity to seek medical help elsewhere. Interestingly, doctors will use this point as the very reason for not telling the truth—they say they hate to see patients pointlessly wasting their money running around to different doctors. But in making this argument, doctors fail to consider the possibility that other physicians might in fact be able to help the patient. But even in those cases where *no* doctor could help, by not informing the patient of his true condition, the physician also deprives the patient of the opportunity to take care of personal and practical matters which should be settled for the sake of the family and the patient's final wishes. Furthermore, by hiding information from the patient and telling it instead to a family member, the physician leads the family into an upsetting collusion of secrecy and dishonesty that probably makes an already difficult situation even more unbearable.

Finally, it is interesting to observe that while most lay persons agree that physicians are often rude and insensitive and likely to cut off anything but the most minimal conversation with their patients, physicians themselves believe that they know their patients well enough to be able to determine what a patient wishes or wishes not to hear. Finally, in the account that follows, we may observe the doctor's assumption that patients are to be treated somewhat like children:

"Honesty is not always the right thing. It can be cruelty. Doctors must make the determination about what a patient can be told. Why ruin someone's last months if they're dying? I've seen a patient told she has cancer roll over and die of depression. There is no point telling someone what's wrong with them if there's nothing you can do about it. If there's a treatment that's one thing, but not if there isn't.

"And even if patients *ask* to be told everything, you shouldn't necessarily listen to them. You can't just tell people things because they say they want to know, because they're curious. Children are curious—they always want to know things—are you going to tell them everything they want to know? No, you don't load up a child with the weight of knowledge and you don't do it to patients either.

"Doctors know when a patient can tolerate information—it's part of our work. We're trained to judge which patient can handle information. I get to know my patients so well that I'm sure I know what I can tell them and what I can't. I can show you my charts. I know *everything* about them—about their most intimate lives . . . whether they're homosexual or if they're sleeping with their wives. . ."

Like admitting to a patient that there is nothing to be done, losing a patient in the operating room may be upsetting to some surgeons more because it exposes them in situations they cannot control than because of the outcome for the patient. As the previous chapters have illustrated, questions of failure and error are often impossible to separate from issues of control. In coming to the end of these chapters on mistakes and struggles over control, a description of one cardiac surgeon by his resident may be contemplated:

"When Dalton loses someone in surgery it's like a personal insult to him. You can actually see him get deflated from his usual grandiose mood. So then he has to do something to puff himself up again. Once when we lost someone in surgery he said, the way he sometimes talks out of the side of his mouth, 'Well, it's too bad old Joe died, but he *did* leave a lot of money to our thoracic service.'

"And the other day he left the operating room all deflated after a patient died, but when he came back to the lounge fifteen minutes later after telling the family, he was all smiles again. You could see that there had been a recrudescence of his ego just because he had talked the family into an autopsy that they didn't want. Getting that consent for a post-mortem made him feel in control of the situation again.

"He came into the lounge all beaming and sat us down so he could give us advice. 'Boys,' he said, 'there is no reason for you to ever lose an autopsy. You just have to anticipate their objections and be ready to argue. Sometimes Jewish people say no, it's against their religion, and then I say, "Oh, no it isn't, I have letters from the three denominations of the Jewish Church that say that autopsies are allowed." And I tell them I'd be happy to show them the letters if they have any doubts.

" 'Or sometimes they'll say, no, it was Joe's last wish that his body be left alone and that he not have an autopsy, and they want to abide by his last wish. So then I say, "You know, I came to know Joe pretty well, too, and he was a very fine man who cared about other people. And I know that he wouldn't have wanted anyone else to suffer the way he did— he was the kind of man who would have wanted to have an autopsy done if he thought it could help other people."

" 'But I'll tell you something, boys. Usually when you tell the family that the patient has died they're not going to put up a fight with you if you ask for an autopsy right away. They don't hear a thing you say, and they'll do whatever you want. As a matter of fact, as long as you speak to them in a soothing monotone you could even say, "Old Joe was no damn good and the most useful thing he could ever have done with his life was to give his body to medical science. Please sign right here on the dotted line." And they will.' "

III

OTHER BACKROOMS OF MEDICINE

7

THE EMERGENCY ROOM

THE EMERGENCY ROOM at Lakeside is both a central station or "capital city" for the rest of the hospital, and a separate world with a distinctive atmosphere and set of customs. It is on the ground floor of Lakeside, located at the center of several well-traveled hospital corridors: one leading to the operating room, another to Radiology and X-Ray, another to the department chiefs' and administrative offices, and another to the parking lot. Because of its location, staff members walk by the Emergency Room several times a day as they make their rounds, and it is frequently here that they stop to talk with one another about what is happening in the rest of the hospital.

Aside from those who pass through, the regular staff of the Emergency Room is made up of the Emergency Room nurses and secretaries, the interns and residents doing an ER rotation, and the private surgeons and physicians who take turns "covering" the Emergency Room. These individuals generally station themselves at or around the nurses' desk, which is located in the very center of the treatment area. During the day, and in the early evening, when the Emergency Room is in its busiest period, patients fill up the waiting room outside and one or two are allowed into the treatment area every few minutes.

A great number of people come to the Emergency Room to find out whether they have sprained a foot or wrist, or broken a bone. Many others come to have wounds cleaned and sutured. Each day several more come to check minor backaches and stiffness after automobile accidents, and many others come with abdominal pain, headaches, chest pains, sore throats, viruses and fevers. Many patients come to the Emergency Room for treatment of whatever illnesses they notice (emergency or not) because they do not have regular private doctors they would go to first; many use the Emergency Room in place of private doctors because their health insurance pays for medical care given in an Emergency Room but not in a doctor's office.

The complaint heard most frequently among the regular staff members of the Lakeside Emergency Room is that members of the public "abuse" the Emergency Room by coming with problems that are not really emergencies. Instead of acknowledging and adjusting to the fact that the community regards the Emergency Room as a walk-in clinic and medical center as well as a place to go for emergencies, the Emergency Room staff maintains its own more restricted view of its proper functions.

Despite their opinions, those who work in the Emergency Room are obliged to examine and treat anyone who comes, whether or not the case actually constitutes an emergency. For one thing, the hospital is liable for lawsuit from anyone who has been turned away and is later shown to have been truly sick and injured because immediate medical care was denied. Pressure on the Emergency Room staff to be pleasant to the public also comes from the administration and department chiefs. They are forever reminding the staff that the Emergency Room is an important point of "public relations" with the community, and that a large share of the hospital's revenue comes from cases treated or received in the Emergency Room. The chiefs believe, furthermore, that if the non-emergency patients are given appointments to show up at the hospital's out-patient clinic, many of these patients would fail to return. Nevertheless, those who work in the Emergency Room still feel resentful about the members of the public who use the Emergency Room for routine problems, and the staff often regards such individuals as selfish, crazy, ignorant or too lazy to call up a private doctor. Members of the Emergency Room staff are resentful primarily because they do not like the way the public expects "service" from them, and because they feel that their specialized talents are not fully used in the routine non-emergency cases. And so, although they are required to receive and treat all of these cases, the ER staff manages in small ways to discourage and create inconveniences for those patients who come for treatment without a true emergency. The tendency to get even with the patient is especially strong at nighttime or during the weekends, when patients are seen to "misuse" the hospital most often.

For example, at about eight o'clock one weekday evening, the following conversation took place between a fifty-year-old man who wished to have his ears cleaned of wax and an irritated Emergency Room nurse:

Man: "I'd like to have my ears blown out."

Nurse: (Obviously annoyed) "You know, that's not the kind of thing that should be done in an Emergency Room. Can't you come to the clinic tomorrow?"

Man: (Smiling) "No, I can't."

Nurse: "You can't?"

Man: (Still smiling) "No, I have to go to work tomorrow."

Nurse: "How long have your ears been bothering you?"

Man: "About a week."

Nurse: "A week. And don't you have a doctor you might have called all week?"

Man: "No."

Nurse: "Well, this isn't really the place to have your ears cleaned."

Man: "Well, I was visiting someone in the hospital and I thought as long as I'm here I might as well come in and take care of it."

Nurse: "Well, you can wait if you want, but it will be *some* time before anyone can see you. There are people here with priority. With illness that requires immediate care."

Man: "About how long, would you say?"

Nurse: "No, I can't say, but about an hour, at least an hour. Maybe two hours, I would say."

Man: (Still hoping to persuade her) "Oh, that long. I thought I would just come in and take care of it."

Nurse: (Snapping and walking away) "Well, you can wait, if you want to."

As soon as the man was out of sight the nurses remarked about what nerve the public had to expect to get instantaneous service on non-emergency problems. In fact, the Emergency Room was very quiet that night and there were no other patients who had to be seen. Still, the staff liked to discourage people from using the Emergency Room as a clinic, and if they could not actually refuse treatment they could make it extremely inconvenient. Since there were no emergencies the intern enjoyed a leisurely dinner in the hospital cafeteria and some of the nurses retired to the lounge for a coffee break before making themselves available to the man with wax in his ears. By the time the intern returned from dinner, the man had left.

In another characteristic incident, on one Saturday afternoon the Emergency Room was particularly busy and the staff surgeon had not had a moment to rest throughout hours of seeing one patient after another. Although he was collecting a nice fee-for-service from each of the patients he saw (a small suture job that took ten minutes of his time might bring him $40, so that each hour in the Emergency Room during the busy time could bring him $200), he had become impatient with fatigue as the afternoon wore on, and especially irritable with those patients who were not very ill.

As he directed one young woman he had examined to the check-out desk he called after her, "By the way, do you know this is an Emergency Room?" After the patient was out of hearing range the delighted charge nurse feigned shock, "Marty! What did you say to one of our patients!" The surgeon walked over to the nurses' desk and complained to the intern, "This girl came in and said she's had a pain in her wrist for three months and wanted to know what's wrong with it. I gave her a thorough work-up. I couldn't find anything wrong with her, so I told her so. So she said to me, 'Thanks a lot.' So I said, 'Do you know this is an Emergency Room?' I know that's the wrong thing to do—I should have explained to her that with a problem like that she could get better treatment by seeing her doctor or going to a specialist. But after seeing thirty patients in a row, something like that comes out. It's only out of hostility I said that. It won't teach her anything."

The intern laughed and was pleased that one of the private doctors was willing to complain about patients with him. "I don't think that was inappropriate. It's more effective to yell at her than to explain anything to her."

The surgeon continued: "Maybe that's true, but I was rough like that all the time when I was younger and I'm not very proud of myself when I'm like that. But maybe you're right. She's the type who will pop right back in here again with something else like that."

The intern repeated, "I don't think it was uncalled for."

The nurse interrupted the conversation to remind the intern that there were five patients waiting to be examined. He replied that he would see them as soon as he finished his conversation. The surgeon later reported that he regretted the conversation, for he didn't want to encourage the house staff to be rude to patients.

The Emergency Room staff is especially likely to get angry with non-emergency patients late at night when the staff is tired and would like to take the rest of the evening easy. One busy evening, a young, married black couple who had come to the Emergency Room complaining of skin rashes were kept waiting for several hours while others who had arrived later were ushered right into the treatment area. The intern on duty that night expressed irritation that the couple wanted to use the Emergency Room as a clinic, and he had decided to keep them waiting a long time in order to make the Emergency Room no more convenient to use than the out-patient clinic. They made no complaints but sat quietly in the waiting room from 8 P.M. until almost 1 A.M. Finally, they were brought into adjacent treatment cots, separated only by a curtain.

The intern was still annoyed with the couple and when the husband showed him the scabs and rashes around his finger joints, the intern asked in a loud voice if he had ever had gonorrhea. The man, lowering his voice (since his wife was sitting on the other side of the curtain), replied in a soft voice that he had gonorrhea when he was in Vietnam but it had been treated.

The intern informed the man, with obvious irritation, that his blood pressure was very high and that he should have it treated at the hospital clinic or by his own doctor. Then he prepared a hypodermic syringe in order to take a blood sample. The man asked nervously, "Is it serious?"

The intern replied, raising his voice to a loud volume again, "Well, your blood pressure could be serious. As for the rash, to be perfectly frank, I'm not a dermatologist so I'm not the one who should be treating this, but the only thing I want to rule out is [he jabbed in the needle] gonorrhea."

The Emergency Room staff is annoyed not only by patients who "abuse" the services by coming with non-emergency symptoms but also by those who they feel should go to another hospital. For example, one evening a young couple arrived at Lakeside and the wife reported that her husband was suffering from abdominal pains. The couple were students from Iran, and the wife, who seemed more familiar with English, did all the talking. They belonged to a health maintenance organization, a prepaid health plan that offered emergency care through a group of hospitals which did not, however, include Lakeside. The nearest hospital included in their insurance plan was a mile away, and they had come to Lakeside because it was closer, and felt that since this was an "emergency" Lakeside should take care of it and bill their own health plan for the costs. An orderly and Irene, the charge nurse, were the first to speak to them and they explained that even if the doctors did the work-up examination at Lakeside, if it turned out that the patient had to be admitted to a hospital he would not be admitted to Lakeside anyway, but would have to be sent to the nearby hospital included in their health plan. So it seemed more appropriate for the patient to be examined in the other hospital.

The wife became excited and waved her health plan membership card in the air, shouting, "You're refusing to see him when he might have a burst appendix? You can't do that. I called them [her health plan] up and they said we could go to any hospital we want."

The argument was turning into a scene with several patients looking on, and so the surgeon "covering" the Emergency Room that night intervened with the excited wife. "Look, calm down. I will personally look at your husband even though I'm not working now." He directed them to a cot but the wife was no longer sure she wanted to stay. The surgeon whispered to the charge nurse, "Irene, call up the administrator and tell him this patient was offered care, so whatever happens we'll be covered."

The wife continued to scream at the nurse from the other end of the corridor, "You have no right to act like an investigator. You're just here to administrate medicine." She held the card up in the air again. "This card is good anywhere."

The surgeon shook his head angrily at the nurse. "She's crazy. Call up University Community Health Plan and tell them there's a crazy person here disturbing our Emergency Room and it's their patient." He turned back to the couple smiling, "Look, we shouldn't be taking care of you. Even though they might have told you that you can go to any hospital, if it turns out that this is *not* an emergency they won't pay us and we never can collect our payments from them."

The wife started shouting, "Oh, so you're worried about the money. We would pay." The surgeon angrily retorted, "No, it's not the money. I just write these off—I'm used to losing my fee on these cases." The couple turned to go, threatening that they would be writing a letter to the administrator about how they were refused emergency care. The surgeon, clearly furious but anxious to avoid an incident, adopted a conciliatory tone: "Look, I didn't know you called your health plan and they said you could come here. I didn't know anything about it. The nurse didn't tell me."

Irene was unwilling to have the blame shifted to *her*, so she added, "Well, don't blame me; it was the orderly's fault. He shouldn't have told you to go somewhere else."

When the couple nevertheless marched out, threatening to write a letter to the administrator, Irene muttered, "You can take that card and shove it up your ass." She was obviously shaken, worrying about whether the administration would punish her for the incident. The surgeon tried to reassure her, "Forget it. She won't do anything. She'll just jabber herself out. A crazy person like that. You can't reason with people like that."

At the times when the Emergency Room was quiet and the staff sat around the desk, waiting for something to happen, they would recount stories to one another about the most bizarre cases that had lately passed through. What they felt to be the "crazy" or "difficult" patients were grouped together in different categories. There were the ordinary "turkeys" who either worried too much about symptoms the doctors considered insignificant or who ignored their significant symptoms for too long a time. Then there were the individuals who phoned the Emergency Room for advice on unusual medical matters: for example, one woman had called to report that she had eaten several petunia flowers and wanted to know whether petunias were poisonous. There were other patients with requests considered odd or inappropriate for an Emergency Room, such as young men who came to have an ear pierced. The staff also talked about patients who offered their own diagnoses of unusual conditions. About these patients the doctors joked that they had watched too many television medical programs, which had turned them into "experts," and lamented how "a little information was a dangerous thing." Patients who had been involved in a violent activity were also viewed as noteworthy: for example, men who came with lacerations incurred in a fight, or women who were hyperventilating because their husbands or boyfriends had yelled at or threatened them.

There were drug addicts who brought false complaints of injury and pain in order to obtain prescriptions for opiates. Often they would deny ever having been in the hospital, and the nurses seemed especially pleased when they recognized these individuals and caught them in the act of lying. On these occasions the nurse would produce the medical record, alerting the staff against believing the patient's story and prescribing drugs, and they would threaten the patients with police arrest if they ever showed up in the Emergency Room again.

There were people who had pushed a ring onto a finger that was too large, and who needed to have the ring cut off because their finger was swelling. There were others who had jammed a ring over other unfortunate spots. Most memorable in this category were stories of a young man who, unable to have an erection during intercourse, had out of desperation pushed his ring over his penis and now needed to have the ring cut off his swollen organ.

Finally, there were cases involving patients who had tried to kill or mutilate themselves, and they frequently provided lively material for staff gossip. The staff was especially uneasy with patients who had tried to commit suicide, and not knowing what to say to these individuals, they would often treat them with anger and hostility.

For example, one night a well-known writer was brought to the Emergency Room after a friend had discovered him collapsed on the floor in his home. The man had been admitted to the hospital a few times in recent months after attempting to commit suicide by swallowing large amounts of sleeping pills.

When he was brought into the Emergency Room practically unconscious, one of the nurses slapped his face a few times, interrogating, "Come on, John. What did you take this time?" The patient, who was having trouble speaking, denied repeatedly that he had taken any drugs but the usual prescription ordered by his physician, and pleaded that he was frightened at lapsing into unconsciousness because he didn't know why it was happening to him. In fact, the patient was later shown to have been telling the truth: he had recently been placed on a prescription of an antidepressant medication for which the therapeutic dose was very close to the toxic dose. But before this information was available, the intern on duty in the Emergency Room expressed obvious annoyance that doctors should have to waste their time on people who wanted to kill themselves, and he told the nurse that he would take a coffee break in the staff lounge before looking at the patient.

The Chief of Surgery happened to come through the Emergency Room that night, and was upset when he discovered that the famous writer had been left unexamined and practically unconscious in the Emergency Room observation room. The patient was by now becoming somewhat more alert and had asked to be helped into the bathroom. The nurse had handed him a bedpan and told him that if he needed the bathroom he could use the bedpan. The Chief of Surgery walked up to the nurses' desk, appalled: "Don't you know who that is? He's one of our greatest living writers." The nurses shrugged off the matter and replied that the chief should complain to the intern who was sitting and reading a magazine in the lounge. As the surgeon stormed off in the direction of the lounge, the nurses laughed at him and complained that they didn't care how great the patient was, he could use the bedpan like everyone else.

One of the distinctive features of the Lakeside Emergency Room was that the nurses were sometimes in the unusual position of being able to assert some authority over the interns: the nurses who had worked in the Emergency Room for a long time often knew a great deal more about emergency medicine than did the new interns fresh out of medical school. Furthermore, the nurses who had worked there for a long time often came to view the Emergency Room as their own territory (much like the operating room nurses) and resented the ways that the new, inexperienced interns (who worked in the ER for only a month or two) tried to throw their weight around. When an intern was not duly respectful of their superior knowledge, the Emergency Room nurses would retaliate by reminding an intern each time he (female interns were generally more respectful of the nurses and did not have these run-ins with them) relaxed that patients were waiting to be seen. An angry nurse would sometimes score a victory by suggesting to an intern that a resident or private doctor be consulted on a case before the intern acted on his own judgment. Such liberties with the strict hierarchy could only be attempted by the nurses during the first few months of the medical year (which began with July). After a few months the new interns became sure enough of themselves not to act respectfully toward, or tolerate any assertiveness from, the nurses. But at least for the first few months, the nurses could enjoy "breaking in" the interns, as they liked to call it. When interns felt that they weren't being treated with sufficient respect they would characteristically ignore the nurses' suggestions, sometimes going so far as to show no indication of having heard the nurses' remarks.

For example, one afternoon a young woman patient who had swallowed a handful of sleeping pills was brought into the Emergency Room and was being treated by her private doctor (one of the senior teaching doctors on the hospital staff), who had drawn the curtain around her bed. The intern was curious to see how the senior doctor was handling the situation, and heading for the bed, he told the nurses where they could find him. The charge nurse explained that the doctor had left word that he and the patient should not be interrupted in their conversation because the patient was extremely upset. The intern, resenting the nurse's interference, retorted, "Well, I'm interested so I'll be looking in on it." The nurse answered that he really shouldn't, the senior doctor had said that the patient was very unbalanced and he wanted to have a private talk with her and handle it himself, and he had come down to the Emergency Room specifically to do that. The intern, unwilling to give in to the nurse, insisted: "Well, I'll just walk by and look in."

This intern had been involved in frequent skirmishes with the nurses, and these culminated one night in a rather dramatic fight. As this final incident illustrates, even private doctors and house officers will usually forget their arguments and differences when it comes to "insubordination" from a nurse.

The intern, Jim Lilly, had been upsetting the nurses all week by repeatedly discouraging patients from using the Emergency Room; the nurses felt that several of these patients might have been seriously ill. To each one, he had suggested that they make an appointment with a private doctor. One young woman who had been turned away (she had been discouraged enough to leave) from the Emergency Room when she complained of abdominal pain (Lilly thought the pain was psychosomatic) had later turned out to have been suffering from an ovarian cyst. Several young women who were suffering from painful pelvic inflammatory disease had been treated rudely by the intern and told to see their gynecologists. The nurses, offended by what they perceived as the intern's arrogance and laziness, had several times asked the various private doctors on call for the serious cases in the ER to intervene in the situation, but they had been reluctant to get involved. One evening, however, the private doctor on call for the Emergency Room had been sitting at the nurses' desk complaining to another doctor (but within the hearing range of the nurses) that one of his patients had been allowed to die in the Coronary Care Unit because the interns hadn't done anything for the patient, and not one of the nurses in the CCU had called him in to intervene in the situation because they were too fearful and insecure to act on their own initiative. He also complained that patients suffering from heart attacks were poorly cared for in the Emergency Room, and argued that the interns shouldn't be left unsupervised in those cases. Shortly after this conversation, he left the Emergency Room to visit some patients on the floors upstairs. The nurses had silently listened to him, sharing his distress about the incompetence of the interns to handle things in the Emergency Room.

Tension had been building up all that evening between Lilly and the nurses. Each time they had asked him to see a patient he had busied himself in a telephone conversation. There was a tremendous backlog of patients waiting for treatment, including one woman in pulmonary edema and struggling to breathe who had been sitting unattended in a treatment room for over two hours. Maxene, the charge nurse, had overheard the private doctor's complaints earlier in the evening, and decided to call him in to have a look at the very ill woman, thereby departing from the usual custom of allowing the *intern* to decide when he felt he needed help from another doctor.

As she was on the telephone asking Dr. Stern to come to the Emergency Room, the intern, who was sitting nearby, asked her what she was doing. Was this a special case, he wanted to know. The nurse burst out that she hoped the other doctor would take care of *all* the cases, since he, Lilly, was not doing a damn thing. The intern angrily departed for the staff lounge. The nurse exploded to the two staff surgeons standing nearby that the intern was a "lazy sonofabitch"; the two doctors ignored her remark and moved away.

In the meantime, while Lilly sat in the lounge, each time a patient asked how much longer it would be before someone examined them, Maxene had to mask her anger and politely apologize that the doctor was very busy and would see them as soon as he could.

When Stern finally arrived in the Emergency Room, Maxene and Jane, another nurse, poured out complaints about how lazy the intern was, and how they could no longer bear to work with him. One of the nurses, near tears, explained that she cried herself to sleep every night thinking about how patients had been badly treated in the Emergency

Room. The intern had now emerged from the lounge, and sucking on his pipe, stood by and listened to the string of complaints about him. At one point he shook his head and explained in an exasperated voice that the nurses simply did not understand that he had been working very hard all night.

Stern looked embarrassed. He had been complaining about the interns only earlier in the evening, but he obviously did not want to take the side of the nurses, when it was very important for him to have the cooperation of the house officers. He looked from the nurses to the intern and uncomfortably agreed, "Yes, I think there *should* be a resident here to work with the intern," but then he put his arm on the shoulder of the intern and the two men walked off together in the direction of the staff lounge. As soon as they turned their backs to the nurses they could be seen laughing and shaking their heads, apparently at the scene the nurses had created.

After Maxene comforted Jane, who was by then sobbing, they silently cleaned up the desk and restocked the linen supplies in each of the treatment areas. Lilly emerged smiling from the staff lounge about ten minutes later and spent the rest of the evening on the telephone, having long conversations with various friends both inside and outside the hospital.

CHAPTER

8

THE REVENGE OF THE NIGHTWORKERS

AFTER NIGHTTIME VISITING hours are over and the hospital is vacated by everyone but the patients and a skeleton night staff, a different mood descends on the wards. With the corridors empty and activity practically at a standstill, even the background sounds are different: the daytime human noises are replaced each night by the mechanical sounds of the night shift. From the darkened patient rooms one can always hear the rhythmic chirps of cardiac monitors, the slow whistling of respirators and the gurgling sounds of bubbles and gases bursting in bottles of fluids. At Lakeside Hospital one could also hear the metallic footsteps of Randy, one of the night shift orderlies, as he walked along the corridors, for he always wore large taps on the toes and heels of his shoes, and the sounds echoed in the empty hallways.

With the departure of the daytime personnel (the teaching and service staff, administrators, department chiefs, attending doctors and most of the house officers), the hospital and its patients were left each night to the care of the lowest status staff members, the nightworkers; and until seven o'clock the following morning this odd assortment of often bizarre-looking and -acting individuals would reign over the vast empires abandoned each night by the daytime supervisors.

The night shift at Lakeside, like that of many twenty-four-hour institutions, had a character all its own, for not only did most of the activities familiar to the daytime come to a stop at night, but the nightworkers who were clustered in little groups around the hospital were distinguished by odd manners, bizarre physical appearances, and noticeable idiosyncracies. The orderly with the tapped shoes was the most sociable of the lot: he would pay visits around the staff lounges and nurses' stations every night in order to report the latest progress on the sportscar he was building from a kit. Then there was a huge charge nurse on the sixth floor; according to others on the night shift, she had never engaged in a friendly conversation during the three years she had been working at the hospital. Night after night, her words were restricted to necessary communications and snapping at anyone who came too close to her desk. There was a Portuguese orderly who carried his portable radio and played music wherever he went, thereby breaking one of the many hospital rules that no one bothered to enforce at night. There was a maid, one of the "mentally retarded" workers the hospital had employed for several years at low wages to do the "housekeeping." She wore bright red lipstick smeared across her lips and ate her dinner alone at a separate table every night in the hospital cafeteria, for no one ever invited her to join them. (There was another "mentally retarded" employee who did the housekeeping in the daytime shift. He had formerly worked in the hospital cafeteria, cleaning up trays and tables, until a few diners had complained that they found his presence objectionable at mealtimes, and so he had been transferred to the floor-mopping service).

In thinking about the world of nighttime one is reminded of the film called *Freaks*, directed by Tod Browning in 1932. It is about a tightly knit society of human freaks who work and live together in a traveling circus. Their world is upset by the intrusion of a glamorous and beautiful trapeze artist and her boyfriend, the circus strongman. The couple deceive the midget man into bequeathing his life savings to the trapeze artist, and soon after, they attempt to poison him. In retaliation, one night, as a violent hurricane rips through the carnival grounds and turns everything into mud, all the freaks emerge from their tents and come sliding through the mud to converge and inflict a terrible revenge on the evil couple: the glamorous pair are turned into freaks themselves.

This motif appears in other kinds of stories. There are tales of ghosts who come out at night to haunt those who hurt them in life. There are children's stories about oppressed or imprisoned figures of the daytime who come to life or who get to enjoy themselves at night: stories of toys that jump off the shelves and take over the toy shop, living the dramas of their own unsuspected societies until the morning breaks when they must return once again to their boxes and places as wooden figures handled roughly and carelessly by the shopowners and customers. In Sigmund Freud's psychoanalytic perspective, as well, the impulses repressed by society in the daytime have their moment at night when they take charge of the mind through dreams.

Like these fictional representations of nocturnal activities, each night Lakeside Hospital sustained a ceremonial and virtual collapse of its daytime social order. The disappearance of the daytime social hierarchy and its rigidly enforced status distinctions was made possible by the departure of all but the lowest status nurses and orderlies. Left without interference from supervisors, the nightworkers could stretch out and rest their feet on the desks of those who ruled the hospital in the daytime. Those nightworkers who were more sociable congregated into little parties, defying the customary solemnity of the hospital with the sounds of their radios. These gatherings were nicely rounded out by policemen who visited the hospital to kill a few hours from *their* night shifts; often when policemen had business in the hospital, such as bringing in an emergency patient, they would stay and visit for a while. Occasionally the policemen brought in pizza pies, and these were sliced and served with the same surgical knives used for more dignified purposes in the daytime.

The nightworkers lived and worked unencumbered by the rules and restrictions that presided over the hospital in the daytime. Unlike the daytime workers, who followed the rules precisely, the nightstaff, for a variety of reasons, seemed to be unconcerned with many of the regulations. Some of the nightworkers regarded their jobs as temporary or secondary work, incidental to their real interests, and they did not take their work as seriously as the daytime personnel, to whom it was a profession. Some, for example, were graduate students, musicians or artists who had chosen their nighttime jobs either to support their daytime activities and identities or because the night provided an opportunity to read and study while drawing wages. These nightworkers refused to submit to the deferential behavior of a subordinate position with which they did not otherwise identify.

Other members of the night shift seemed socially "unregulated" for other reasons. Some did not speak English and were therefore only tenuously connected to the social network of the hospital and its code of behavior. Others displayed an obvious preference for being left entirely alone, and some were markedly physically unattractive by conventional standards: either unusually tall or short or misshapen. Their appearances punctuated their social marginality.

The hospital is a world of extreme differences in social status. In the same room one finds surgeons, who are treated practically like gods, along with practically unnoticed janitors and maids. Like their daytime counterparts (the orderlies and aides) and the mentally retarded workers, the nightstaff was practically invisible to the high-status daytime staff. And although the hospital prided itself on being good to its low-status workers (the head of the nursing department boasted: "Those employees complain that we are inhuman to them but I'm even friendly with a big black guy who supervises the laundry service and every effort is made to make them feel like persons. It's just not true that this place is inhumane. Last week, Iris, a maid who cleaned these administrative offices, was leaving the hospital and she was given a coffee hour which even the administrators came to and she was given presents and you'd think she was in administration, the way she was treated. So it's just not true that people here are treated badly"), the nightworkers were glad to be working when no one would order them around.

Even those few interns or residents who were "on" at night

would behave differently than they did in the daytime. Giddy and light-headed with fatigue from working through thirty-six hours with little or no sleep, many would display uncharacteristic friendliness toward the orderlies and nurses, thereby joining in the suspension of status distinctions.

One surgical resident, a very gentle and philosophical doctor from Greece, seemed never to get to sleep at all. Whenever he was on night call (which was every third night) he would quietly pad around all the wards in his slippers, dragging his feet more and more wearily as the night wore on, until it was time to shave and shower for six-thirty morning rounds. His partner, a surgical intern who was more eager to get to bed for a few hours, would nonetheless, out of loyal friendship, stay up through the night with the resident and listen to long soliloquies about the nature of the soul and the masochism of doctors. The resident had affectionately nicknamed the intern "The Prince" and the intern called the resident "Professor." This pair of surgical house officers were favorites among both the nurses and the patients, for they had somehow managed, unlike many of the other residents, to retain their emotional responsiveness and personal liveliness despite the exhausting ordeal of their long hours. In their concern for the patients they were exceptions to the general atmosphere of indifference that prevailed in the night hours.

However much one might appreciate the nightly collapse of overly rigid rules and formalities and applaud the symbolic revenge of the nightworkers, it is nonetheless disturbing to consider the nighttime situation from the patient's point of view. Indeed, patients often come to realize that the nighttime is the wrong time to be in need. But the problem is not restricted to the fact that patient calls may go unanswered for long periods at night. More serious is the problem that the largest share of nursing mistakes is likely to occur during the night shift. At least at Lakeside Hospital it appeared that it was during the night shift that the wrong medications were most often given, or drugs given in the wrong doses, that orders on patient care were most frequently overlooked or forgotten, and that serious changes in patients' conditions most often went unnoticed.

When nursing supervisors talk about the problems of mistakes and incompetence during the night shift they often claim that there is nothing they can do, since few of the most experienced nurses are willing to work at night. They explain that in order to cover the night shift at all they must take what nurses they can get. Some hospitals and wards, however, maintain a policy of requiring all daytime nurses to take an occasional night shift, thereby insuring some uniformity in the quality of staff coverage across the shifts. Still, even those staff members who normally follow the rules carefully in the daytime are likely to be a bit more lax at night. Although in general the night shift offers the worst care for patients, there are occasional nightworkers who are unusually considerate of patients' needs; indeed, they choose the night shift partly because it offers more time and freedom to deal with patients in a personal way. But as most of the following illustrations suggest, the nighttime is a period of increased difficulty for patients.

At Lakeside Hospital one winter there was a severe rash of thefts from patients' rooms—mainly occurring during the night hours, and probably committed by a staff member. In the dark of the night, watches and wallets from the patients' bedside tables were vanishing in large numbers. Each time a theft was reported an "incident report" had to be submitted by the nursing staff to the administrator. In characteristic fashion, the patients were blamed for their misfortunes, even when the incident involved a theft, as the following incident report illustrates: "When patient went to sleep she placed her watch and purse in her bedside table, and when she awoke her watch and forty dollars from her purse were missing. Patient was told not to keep valuables at bedside, and stated that she knows it was wrong to do so." (Incident reports are also submitted when a medication or treatment order has been mixed up or overlooked; included in the report is a list of persons who are aware of the mistake, as well as an indication of whether the patient is aware that something went wrong.)

Frequently a patient in distress would realize that there was little help available during the night hours. For example, a man hospitalized for asthma paced the hospital corridors all one night in extreme agitation and near tears until the daytime staff arrived at seven o'clock the following morning. He had dreaded an incipient asthma attack but the nurse had been unable to give him any medication for relief of his breathing difficulties without the authorization of the intern covering the floor that night. The intern had refused to get out of bed to examine the patient because he believed that the man's anxiety about suffocating was caused by a neurotic syndrome that he (the intern) did not care to indulge.

Violations of professional decorum that would probably not be tolerated in the daytime often go unnoticed in the night shift. One respiratory therapist, for example, when administering treatment to patients in the Intensive Care Unit, would pull the curtains around the beds of attractive young women patients and with little chance of any resistance from the patients (for they had undergone cardiac surgery only hours or days before) would enjoy various degrees of sexual trespass. One teen-aged girl (who was sexually inexperienced but noticeably flirtatious) who had undergone heart surgery reported the following story: "The respiratory therapist would draw the curtains shut and kiss me when I was in the Intensive Care Unit. I didn't mind when it was just little pecks on my cheek but then he started to give me deep kisses and he asked me whether I was feeling well enough to make love. I said to him, 'What makes you think I indulge?' "

The experience of one woman who was moved into the post-surgical ward late one night following abdominal surgery also illustrates some of the special dangers the nighttime brings for patients:

Ellen Freund had undergone a long abdominal operation. Her surgery, begun at 3 P.M., had taken more than five hours to complete, and she was moved from the recovery room to her new private room on the post-surgical floor after 11 o'clock one night. As she was transferred into her bed she felt incapable of moving and was increasingly aware of a sharp pain on her side, where the surgical incision had been made. She asked the nurse if she could have something for the pain and the nurse left the room, the patient assumed, in order to get the drug. What seemed to be an hour passed by and the nurse did not reappear. Meanwhile, the pain became severe and the patient called for a nurse again. The same nurse returned and stood silently in the doorway. The nurse was from India and since she once again did not respond to questions, Ellen Freund began to wonder whether the nurse could speak English.

The patient was trying to orient herself after the surgery: she was wondering what time of night it was and how much time had passed since she had been brought to the room. Her disorientation was aggravated by the fact that she had never been in that room before, and so her clock had not been plugged into the wall. The nurse stood staring at her silently. Even after Ellen asked what time it was the nurse made no gesture of response.

Having received no answer the patient complained that she was in severe pain and wanted a pain killer. This time the nurse shook her head no and started to leave the room. Ellen Freund began to feel alarmed at this point. The room was completely dark and there seemed to be no way of getting help from anyone. She was unable to move from the pain and exhaustion she felt. Angrily she shouted out once again that she would like something for the pain. The nurse shook her head no and pointed to her watch and finally spoke, "No, it's not time. Not time. You have to wait."

The patient asked, "Well, what time is it? And what time can I get the drug? I just want to know." The nurse shook her head and started to walk out the door. The patient called out after her, hoping someone else might hear and intervene, "How long do I have to wait, I asked you? Can't you answer a question?" The nurse angrily replied, "An hour and a half," and left the room.

Ellen felt despair. To go an hour and a half more with her pain seemed unimaginable, and she felt that she had been left in the care of a crazy woman. After a few minutes the door swung open again, letting in the bright light from the corridor into the dark room. The nurse was back, aiming a flashlight in Ellen's eyes. She had brought a bedpan and was telling Ellen that she had to use it, immediately. Ellen Freund didn't feel any impulse to urinate and so she shook her head no. The nurse dropped the pan on the bed and, pulling back the sheets, began to press on the patient's bladder. "Yes, you have to go. If you don't use the bedpan we'll have to put a catheter in."

Ellen was beginning to feel desperate, but she tried to command the woman away. She was in extraordinary pain and the thought of the catheter made her want to cry, but she resisted the nurse. "No, I don't have to go and I don't want a catheter put in. Just leave me alone." There was already a nasogastric tube running from her nose into her stomach, connected to a suctioning machine beside her bed that was drawing out all the gastric juices from her stomach. Another tube, which had been inserted into her bile duct came through her body via the surgical incision and emptied bile into a bottle placed on the floor near her bed. There was an intravenous line running into the veins of her right hand, stomach, connected to a suctioning machine beside her bed Now, in all this pain, attached to all these devices and being threatened by a nurse who appeared to be insane, Ellen decided she would not allow any urinary catheter to be inserted, and she wondered if they would try to force or restrain her.

The nurse had left to get the intern and now she returned with a slight, gentle-looking young man, barely visible in the dark room. Now *he* began to press on the patient's bladder, with the nurse gesticulating angrily from behind. Ellen Freund was relieved to see another person and hoped he would be more reasonable. "I don't have to urinate. I don't want a catheter." Still pressing around her bladder, he answered, "You wouldn't be able to feel it even if your bladder were full, because you won't have any sensations there for a few days. We can't let your bladder get distended, but it does feel all right to me now." He turned to the nurse, "She doesn't need a catheter now. She's not distended."

They left the room again and Ellen was relieved. But the nurse returned again a few minutes later and started to press on her bladder once more. Ellen Freund was worried. She knew she couldn't use the bedpan, especially with this woman standing over her. Finally, to get rid of the nurse, she said she would try to use the toilet.

The nurse should not have allowed the patient to drag herself across the room to the bathroom only a few hours after surgery, but she had apparently become determined to make the patient empty her bladder. So, disconnecting the NG tube from the suctioning device, and attaching the bile bottle to the bottom of the IV pole, the nurse silently watched the patient wince and moan as she spent twenty minutes dragging herself up into a sitting position with her legs over the side of the bed. She had pulled herself up with her arms clutching the side of the bed rails. The nurse had roughly offered to help her, grabbing on her arm, but Ellen had feared that the nurse would jerk her up so quickly that her abdomen would split open, so she had screamed that she would do it herself. It took her another ten minutes to edge her feet down to the floor. Each slight movement was incredibly painful and she had to rest every few seconds, gasping from pain after every small effort to move off the bed.

She leaned on the stomach pump as she stood on her feet, and grasped furniture along the room as she dragged herself to the bathroom. The nurse followed behind, rolling the IV pole in back of the patient. The bedpan had been placed inside the toilet bowl so that the urine output could be measured. Ellen slowly eased into the toilet seat but still felt no impulse to empty her bladder. The nurse stood watching her, saying she would have to empty her bladder or go back to bed and have a catheter inserted. The patient screamed at the nurse to go away, and when the woman finally left the room, Ellen sat sobbing on the toilet seat.

The nurse returned every few minutes, standing by the bathroom with her arms folded. Ellen had slammed the bathroom door shut. After sitting up, extremely dizzy, for over two hours, Ellen finally managed to produce a small amount of urine and she dragged herself back to bed.

When the nurses were changing shifts early the next morning, even from her bed, Ellen could hear the night nurse telling the day shift nurses in the hall that the new patient was a real bitch.

When her doctor came around a little later she told him that she was in great pain and asked if he could increase the dosage of pain killer (since the nurse had refused to respond to her complaints of pain on the grounds that she could not exceed the doctor's orders). The doctor smiled and remarked that she must be extremely sensitive to pain to need more than the ordinary prescription. But when he looked at the chart he noticed that the patient had been given less Demerol than he had specified in his orders. He had prescribed 75 to 100 milligrams of Demerol every 3 to 4 hours, and the nurse, perhaps out of anger, had administered only 75 milligrams in more than 4 hours. Returning to the patient, he did not let on what he had discovered. Instead he smiled and said, "Well, since you don't tolerate pain very well, I'll tell you what I'll do. I'll increase your allowance of Demerol." Then he noted in the chart that the patient should be allowed the full amount that he had ordered from the start.

9

THE ENACTMENT OF TRUST: CARDIAC SURGEONS AND PATIENTS

JUST AS MEDICAL mistakes are systematically neutralized (covered up, ignored, made little of, or justified) by doctors who work together, so does patient anger and mistrust go through a similar process of redefinition. There is collusion in every aspect of hospital routine to ignore patient mistrust and to undermine and cool out patient anger, for the direct expression of these feelings (like the open recognition of mistakes) is highly disruptive to the comfort, schedule and convenience of the medical staff. Patients and their families usually offer no resistance to this carefully engineered neutralization of doubt and anger. Since they feel they have little choice or control over their medical treatment or over what is going to happen to them in the hospital, they prefer, like the medical staff, to avoid acknowledging their doubts in the hope that the less mistrust expressed, the less will be experienced. Indeed, they fear (often with good reason) that unless they are uncritical and undemanding, they run the risk of receiving worse treatment from angry physicians and nurses.

The "backrooms" of medicine, then, refer not only to the places and events that are off-limits to patients, but also to the thoughts and subjects of conversation that are avoided, and the emotional expressions that are not allowed in the doctor–patient or even patient–family relationships. And though these expressions are carefully held in check, they often threaten to break through the social conventions and disrupt the situation. The most upsetting ones have to do with indications of mistrust.

The patient's experience is one familiar to other situations: in many relationships and associations (with friends, spouses, work partners) an individual frequently finds that he must act as if he fully trusted, and felt trusted by, the other individual, for the relationship would be disrupted and mutual action become impossible if the actual mistrust were fully and openly acknowledged. Feelings of trust and mistrust are not simply states of mind that an individual is allowed to experience according to his own preference or temperament, for the expression of mistrust is much too disruptive to social encounters to be allowed such free latitude. Like behavior, feelings are shaped by social conventions and etiquette, and the expression of anger and mistrust comes under such strict social regulation that people are often forced to publicly display trust and confidence when they privately feel most doubtful and apprehensive.

Considering the magnitude of what is at stake, patients are exceedingly successful in masking whatever doubts about their doctors they may have acknowledged to themselves. Still, expressions of mistrust inevitably slip through, or are carefully phrased in indirect or unserious manners, and these expressions must be neutralized in order to prevent them from upsetting and dominating the interaction.

The situation of patients undergoing open heart surgery provides a dramatic illustration of the social neutralization of doubt and mistrust that can be found in ordinary conversations among doctors, patients and families. Although the interaction is orchestrated primarily by the physicians, it is enacted by all of the parties involved, each for their own different reasons.

It is not surprising that patients would wish to ignore their own mistrust. There are times in life when a sense of safety is maximized by ignoring danger in the environment. Sometimes openly showing what one has noticed may subject the observer to further risk (as in the case of the sleeper who awakens to discover a burglar). Sometimes admitting to knowledge may force the individual into public stands or actions that he or she would prefer to avoid (as in the case of the individual who discovers a spouse's extramarital affairs). Finally, as the stock character of the rejected lover always discovers, people are most foolishly trusting and recklessly blind to signs of danger when they want something badly. All of these considerations enter into the situation of surgical patients.

Most of the patients undergoing heart surgery are under the impression (correct or not) that there is little or no choice about their operations. By and large, their surgeons tell them that they have a choice of either refusing surgery and living only a short time (a few months, a few years) with considerable discomfort, or alternatively, of taking a relatively "small" risk in undergoing heart surgery. Since surgical consent forms are designed to protect the doctor and hospital from lawsuit rather than to insure that the patient has full information, the dangers of the operation are made to appear as small as possible. For example, mortality rates that are quoted may reflect the likelihood of death in the operating room but exclude the expectable proportions of surgery-related deaths in the weeks following the operation. Under the circumstances, very few patients refuse to undergo the surgery since the alternative appears so unattractive. Frequently, since they see no choice they would just as well ignore their doubts and misgivings. Like the sleeper who hears strange noises in the house, they figure they are more likely to come through the situation successfully if they ignore suspicious clues and sleep through the experience. Patients are encouraged in this avoidance by hospital staff members who communicate the notion that the "good" patient is the one who asks the fewest questions.

Friends and family members, for their part, feel that it is their special duty to cheer up the patient and help him or her to adjust to the operation and post-surgical "discomforts." With a strained but determined tone of optimism, daily visitors exhort the patient to "listen to the doctor for your own good" and join the hospital staff in discounting or making light of the patient's worries, thereby leaving little room and no social validation for the expression of the patient's anger and mistrust.

Doctors and staff members have the most to gain from the outward display of patient trust and the cloaking of suspicion or doubts. Paying attention to direct or indirect signs of nervousness and mistrust requires a great deal of doctor time and energy, and may make the doctor more vulnerable to uneasy feelings should the surgery go badly. Furthermore, by neutralizing signs of patient mistrust, the surgeon can sustain a more pleasant and amiable atmosphere in his patient contacts.

A display of "trust" by a patient for his surgeon is not, then, an automatic response that wells out of the individual's innermost feelings. Trust, rather, is a dramatic effect produced by the constant, unremitting efforts of everybody concerned to head off, ignore, and if necessary, neutralize the expression of disturbing thoughts. These efforts are expended in several strategic lines of action: they are built, first of all, into the background setting and etiquette of patient-staff contacts and the careful censorship of information that works to prevent the recognition and expression of mistrust. Should this fail, there is a second line of defense: an assortment of expressive techniques for minimizing or neutralizing patient mistrust once it has broken through the social barriers and been experienced or displayed.

An "atmosphere" of safety and trust is introduced by the outward manners of the staff and doctors: physicians present themselves and their surgical proposals with an air of confidence and certainty, and doctors and staff make up a "united front" in support of the procedure being recommended and of one another's expertise. They refrain from showing any doubts or disagreements about the treatment to the patient, and praise one another to the patient (whatever their private assessments may be). Nurses likewise routinely assure the patient that the surgeon is "one of the best" and that patients come from "all over the country" to have this particular surgeon and be in this particular hospital. Then, if a patient should entertain a doubt about a particular doctor, the suspicion is undermined by the belief that if the hospital is so good, so must be each of the doctors. Friends and family members also typically join the staff in singing the praises of the hospital and discounting patient concerns. For example, when one patient expressed doubts to her husband about agreeing to heart surgery, the husband teased her: "Come on, don't make such a fuss about it. These guys do it every day. It's nothing for them."

The first and most obvious technique for insuring "trust" is to keep the patient from hearing any disturbing information once it is known that he will probably consider or undergo surgery. Tales of success and of dramatic improvement following surgery are recounted to the patient. Reassuring visits to the patient might even be paid by members of the Mended Hearts Society, a national club composed of former heart surgery patients who give living testimony to the benefits of the operation. The enthusiastic attitude of these visitors toward surgery is insured by the organization's requirement that they go through a training certification process in order to gain permission to pay visits to prospective surgical patients. In their training they are explicitly instructed to "forget any unpleasant incidents" they may remember about their own surgery while paying visits as members of Mended Hearts. Those who cannot be completely counted upon to censor unpleasant information are told that they are not yet ready to make visits, for their "hearts are still mending."

Family members will usually hide their own doubts from the patient, but occasionally a patient will have to screen himself from a nervous relative. For example, several male patients undergoing cardiac surgery left instructions that their wives were to stay away from the hospital and even refrain from telephoning them in the final days before the operation. After surgery, they allowed their wives only a limited number of visits to the hospital. These men complained that their wives "made them nervous," almost to the point of making it impossible for them to undergo the operation. One such patient reported that a year earlier his wife had made him so apprehensive that he cancelled the operation just a few hours before it was scheduled to take place. Since that time he had suffered an additional heart attack and felt that he now had to submit to the operation. Fearing that a visit from his wife would create the same change of mind in the last moments, he had forbidden his wife to communicate with him in any way. Similarly, many patients dread the thought of seeing their spouses or children just before they are to be taken to the operating room. They fear that at the last moment their relatives will be unable to disguise their anxiety, and that the obviousness of their worry will force them, the patients, to finally experience the full depth of their own doubts and concerns.

Despite everyone's efforts to screen out alarming information, various disturbing elements invariably intrude on the patient's attentions and disrupt the "trust" that has been so carefully developed. Disturbances to "trust" come from many sources: unexpected complications or bad experiences in the hospital, disappointing behavior on the part of the doctors, alarming information from the environment, signs that the doctor or family members are not saying all they know. All of these upsetting intrusions challenge the outward appearance of trust and safety which everyone has gone to such care to produce, and the patient will often have to "neutralize" these signals in order to reinstate his own confidence and faith in his surgical care.

For example, patients who are waiting to undergo heart surgery are often placed in the alarming situation of wondering why another patient has failed to return to the ward even days after an operation. Since all the heart surgery patients in one hospital, both preoperative and postoperative, were kept together on one floor (except for the first twenty-four hours after surgery, which were spent in the Intensive Care

Unit), when a patient failed to return to the ward within a few days after surgery there was good reason for the other patients to believe that the patient had either suffered serious complications that kept him in the Intensive Care Unit or, still worse, had died. Since cardiac surgery patients on the ward generally kept careful observations about each other's progress and passed news among themselves about all the cases, it was quite a feat for them to ignore the disappearance of a patient after surgery. Those still awaiting their operations were especially hard-pressed to account for these failures to return. At these times, there was remarkably little inquiry into the absence. If the subject was broached at all, the patients typically reassured one another that the missing patient must have been sent to another floor, even though they had been clearly informed that all cardiac surgery patients were kept in the same ward.

Such a response illustrates a common neutralizing technique of "redefining" the alarming cues in order to give them less upsetting meanings. An interesting example of this process occurred one day when the patients on the cardiac surgery ward heard on the television news that a young, well-known singer had died in heart surgery. Few patients made mention of the event, and those who did agreed that the singer must have been *very* sick (sicker than they were) not to have survived the operation.

Sometimes alarming information about the carelessness of the hospital staff will press itself upon a patient's attention. At about ten o'clock one night a patient who was recovering from heart surgery was exercising by walking up and down the corridor of the hospital wing designated for the special intensive monitoring of post-surgical patients. There were several lights shining over patient doors, indicating that these patients had called for a nurse, but not a single nurse was to be found at the desk or on the floor. Through an opening in the door to the nurses' lounge the patient observed that all of the nurses were crowded into the lounge, enjoying a farewell party for one of the nurses who was leaving the hospital.

Disturbed that all of the nurses were seemingly out of range of patient call signals, the patient "redefined" the alarming sign by commenting that the nurses must have had a "lightboard" in their lounge so they could know when a patient was in need.

In addition to "redefining" the situation, another common technique of neutralizing the feelings and expression of mistrust involves the use of humor. It has often been observed that humor is used to express thoughts that cannot be stated directly. When patients make "jokes" about their anger or mistrust, they manage to give some small recognition to their doubts and criticisms, yet simultaneously keep them carefully in check by presenting these concerns as "not really serious."

Sometimes joking may be combined with redefining the situation. One patient who had undergone coronary artery bypass surgery was upset that he had not yet met his surgeon. Before his surgery took place he had consoled himself over not meeting the surgeon with the thought that he *had* met and liked his cardiologist. He explained that even though he had not met the surgeon, as long as the cardiologist was "on the team" (though he had been told the cardiologist would not be in the operating room) he had confidence in the surgery. After the operation he admitted that he was still disappointed when the surgeon failed to come by but he felt that he could not directly express his disappointment or request a visit. He decided, instead, to make "a little joke" to his cardiologist in the hope that the underlying meaning would be understood and communicated to the surgeon. When he next saw his cardiologist he remarked, "Well, I sure will be embarrassed when I go back to Omaha and everyone asks me how I liked my surgeon and I'll have to say I never met him." The cardiologist expressed surprise that the surgeon had never stopped by and suggested that some unusual circumstance must have interfered with his customary preoperative visit. The patient's strategy was unsuccessful and, in fact, the surgeon never did visit the patient. By the last day of his hospital stay the patient was so disappointed not to have met the surgeon that he redefined events in order to make them less disturbing: he announced that he now believed that one of the young doctors who made daily rounds in the early morning hours was not just another resident but actually his surgeon who had been visiting him every day. Indeed, although the morning visitor in question was actually just another resident, there was some ironic truth in the patient's self-delusion, for the resident had done a much greater part of the operation than had "his surgeon," who was in the operating room during only a small portion of the total surgery.

It is impossible to think about the question of trust and mistrust without considering the extent to which patients "monitor" the environment for danger and observe what is going on around them. Most doctors act as if they assume that patients are thoroughly trusting and that they do not hear, see, think about or notice anything which is not directly addressed to them. From the doctor's point of view, the advantage of making this assumption is that they can conveniently talk in front of patients while making rounds without having to include the patient in their remarks or concern themselves with what the patient might have heard and understood from their conversation. Usually the patients will cooperate with the doctor's treatment of them as insensate by "pretending" not to listen to conversations which do not include them. Thus, while doctors on rounds discuss a patient's case as if the patient were "not present" (for example, by speaking about the patient in the third person even as they touch the patient's body), the patient will often politely remain silent or even cast his eyes upward toward the ceiling or away from the doctors in order to indicate that he is not eavesdropping on a conversation he has not been invited to join. But even when a patient indicates that he has heard what has been said, doctors will frequently persist in their treatment of the patient as an unobservant figure.

For example, one day the thoracic team was making rounds and stopped by the bed of a patient who had been returned to the operating room for repeat operations twice after her original mitral valve replacement surgery. She had required the two subsequent operations because she suffered from excessive post-surgical bleeding which had to be stopped. Since these two reoperations had occurred within a twenty-four-hour period after the original surgery, it was unclear whether the patient remembered any of these complications. Standing around the bed, the chief asked the resident how long it had been since her operation. The resident cryptically answered, "Three weeks since her third op." The chief replied, "Let's try to do it all in one step next time, shall we, gentlemen?" (meaning the residents should be more careful in suturing together the heart). As they turned to leave, the patient, who until now had been listening quietly, asked, "What did you say?" The chief paused and smiled and kept walking out the door. The patient repeated the question to the intern who was trailing behind and still close to her bed. The intern smiled and answered, "He said you're doing very well."

Occasionally one of the senior cardiac surgeons at Lakeside would ignore the customary professional courtesy of hiding mistakes from the patient, and would criticize subordinate staff members for mistakes directly in front of patients. By treating the symbolic social membrane that divided doctors from patients as an actual physical barrier he assumed that since the argument did not include the patient, the patient would not hear the dispute. One day, while examining a patient's surgical wound (which had been purposely left open to allow for drainage after an infection had developed), this surgeon was annoyed to find that the nurses had been using small-sized sponges (bandages) on the open wound. Calling them around the patient's bed, he yelled that they were to use only *large* sponges since the small ones could easily get lost in the gaping wound. After dismissing the nurses, he swiftly departed, while the patient was left to silently worry about still one more danger in a postoperative course that had already been filled with serious complications. The patient could not even give voice to his new alarm, since he was attached to a respirator inserted into his throat, making speech impossible. Indeed, such conversations seem to be held most often in front of intubated patients, perhaps precisely because they are unable to speak. For just as blind persons with normal hearing are often shouted at as if they were also deaf, so are patients, unable to speak because they are intubated, often treated by doctors as if they are also blind and deaf.

Indeed, patients are so thoroughly expected to be non-observant that the rare occasions in which they indicate their watchfulness often seem comical and incongruous. For example, when patients have been given local rather than general anesthesia for an operation, their serious remarks about the operation or their attempts to take part in doctors' conversations as the surgery is underway often bring the staff to laughter.

The humor emerges partly from the fact that the patient's remarks are sober yet "unscientific," but these situations have a comic aspect primarily because there is something incongruously funny about a patient speaking up and making mistrustful observations as the surgery is actually proceeding. Here the patient becomes both a passive object and an active subject at one and the same moment, and the juxtaposition is so extreme as to be humorous.

Thus one surgical team could not restrain from laughing as the patient sagely observed, "I guess you can't smoke in the operating room because you keep a lot of ozone in here." The anesthesiologist, with tears of laughter in his eyes, mockingly agreed, "Oh yes, sir, we always keep the operating room *filled* with ozone." Another surgical team broke into knowing smiles as one alarmed surgical patient (who had been given spinal anesthesia to block sensation in his right leg) kept moaning and insisting that the doctors had made a mistake and were operating on the wrong leg.

Still another example of the unexpectedness and incongruity of patient watchfulness is the following. On the evening before surgery, an anesthesiologist and his intern-assistant paid a visit to a patient in order to make a final check on the patient's condition and to inquire about allergies and explain what would happen the next day. While examining the patient, the anesthesiologist asked about various body scars that indicated previous surgery. When he was done with his questions he asked the patient, "Now is there anything that you would like to ask me?" The patient, treating the doctor's invitation literally, replied, "Yes, what's that growth you have over your lip? Is that a mole, or a wart, or what?" The physician was mildly stunned to have the roles reversed and asked, "What?" The patient repeated his question. Glancing to the intern to smile at how "inappropriate" this question was, the anesthesiologist answered, "Oh, this? It's just a polyp. I've had it all my life and it's completely harmless, although there are a few surgeons who would like to get their hands on it." The patient continued, "Well, you should have it removed." The doctor smiled carefully, "Well, if you have no questions [implying that the patient's question was not a "real" one], I'll be going." As they walked out, the two doctors could be seen shaking their heads.

An interesting exception to the usual lack of appreciation by surgeons of the patient's observing capacities involved the case of a patient who was himself a physician. Immediately following cardiac surgery, the anesthesiologist and cardiologist noticed that the physician-patient had a very rapid heartbeat, which was hard to explain in view of his general condition. When they asked the patient to move his arms and legs and there was no response, they suspected that the patient was still paralyzed from the muscle relaxant that had been used as part of the anesthesia. After some speculation about the possible alternative explanations for the rapid beat, they decided that since the patient was a physician and knowledgeable about the operation and its risks, his rapid heartbeat might have been the result of anxiety from mistaking his temporary paralysis caused by the anesthesia for permanent paralysis due to damage done to the brain during surgery (and being paralyzed he would be unable to speak and communicate his concern). One of the doctors told the other of a case reported in a medical journal of a physician-patient who had erroneously made this same interpretation about his paralysis following surgery, and who had suffered a cardiac arrest (which later proved to be fatal) from the unnecessary anxiety. The two doctors in this case therefore decided to administer a drug that would sedate the doctor-patient enough to make him unconcerned if indeed he were suffering from this worry. What is significant about this case is the fact that it is only when the surgical patient is himself a doctor that the physicians are likely to speculate about what the patient might be thinking about his inability to move. Obviously, even a non-physician might be alarmed to find himself paralyzed following surgery and unable to speak to learn the reason why, but this possibility was never raised with the other patients, who were presumed not be worrying about their conditions.

When patients are treated and expected to act as if they are not observant about their condition or treatment, the assumption has many implications. For the patient it creates a further restriction on the legitimacy of expressing doubts or objections about his or her medical care. For the doctor, it is the first protection against having to pay attention to complaints or disappointments. For, if attempts to screen out alarming information and the patients' efforts to ignore, redefine or joke about their concerns are not sufficient to inhibit the recognition and expression of mistrust, then the neutralization process will arrive at its final phase: the doctor's techniques for making as little as possible out of the patient's expressed concerns. Clearly, the doctor's first strategy for neutralizing mistrust or resistance is simply to ignore it.

Treating the patient as if he weren't present and aware is only the most dramatic form of ignoring patient alarm. By routinely making bedside visits short and hurried, the doctor not only protects his time but also makes it practically impossible for the patient to introduce a serious discussion of worries, objections and concerns. Instead, the patient's alarm may only be voiced in more general and indirect questions which the doctor is free to interpret in terms of their most limited and technical meanings.

For example, one man of forty-two who suffered from severe coronary artery disease was told that his condition was very grave and that he would need to have several bypass grafts inserted into his coronary arteries. What he was not told was that his condition was so poor that he did not actually stand a very good chance of surviving the operation. His surgeon would be using a device called an intra-aortic-balloon-pump to support his circulation during the operation (a form of mechanical assistance sometimes used in the poorest-risk cases). Instead of indicating how poor were his chances (40 percent) of surviving the operation, the surgeon told the patient that the usual mortality risk of the surgery was not large but that since his case was more difficult and risky than many they would have to use an intra-aortic-balloon-pump to compensate for his poor condition. The patient, who was not fully convinced that he wanted the operation, asked, "Will the balloon mean my risk of dying is greater?" The patient was obviously referring to his total chances, with the help of the balloon, of surviving the operation compared to the average survival expectancy. The surgeon, however, chose to interpret the question literally. He answered, "No, the balloon will improve your chances." The doctor thereby allowed the patient (who did, in fact, die in the surgery) to draw a falsely optimistic inference.

Just as the doctor may interpret and answer patient questions in such ways as to minimize the opportunities for patient resistance, so do doctors frequently "redefine" patient remarks in ways that neutralize the implicit mistrust being conveyed. The following incident, involving a postoperative patient, illustrates how doctors may selectively interpret a patient's remarks in order to ignore mistrust.

On the day he was to be discharged from the hospital following cardiac surgery a patient remarked to the surgical residents (who had come by on rounds and were about to leave), "It's all right for me to drive my car now, isn't it?" A resident answered, "No, you shouldn't drive for at least three weeks. You might get into a situation where you couldn't move quickly enough to turn the wheel or respond to something." The patient, apparently upset that this advice would not have been automatically offered had he not asked, replied with irritation: "Well, it's a good thing I asked, isn't it?" The resident, slightly annoyed, repeated once again the reason for not driving. The patient repeated twice more that it was a good thing he had asked. After they left the room the residents offered the explanation that by his remarks the patient meant that he was sorry he asked if he could drive, since in the residents' view he wanted to get away with taking a vacation while on sick leave from work. By not responding to the more obvious interpretation that the patient was angry and upset with *them* for not having advised him on postoperative restrictions, the residents avoided having to deal with an unpleasant situation.

Finally, a doctor may "redefine" and thereby neutralize expressions of a patient's alarm or doubts about surgery or hospital care by discounting them as "normal" and "expectable." Just as the last-minute doubts of prospective brides and grooms are cheerfully dismissed by friends and relatives as natural, unserious and even amusing, so is the doubting patient assured that his thoughts and feelings are due to "natural nervousness" rather than to any real fault with the medical staff. In fact, cardiac surgery patients are often warned that they may at times feel suspicious of their care, or fear that a staff member is going to hurt them, but that if they have these experiences they should remember that these are "normal" feelings which follow surgery and that they will eventually disappear. On the nurse's checklist of preoperative duties, such an "explanation of normal feelings" to the patient is often included along with other routine duties such as preoperative shaving and preparation. This advance warning to the patient is probably reassuring at times. Still, the custom illustrates just how systematically the neutralization of mistrust is built into patient care.

In addition to leaving little time for and ignoring or redefining signs of patient mistrust, doctors frequently neutralize these expressions by making jokes about them and treating them as unserious. For example, when a patient directly indicated mistrust for her doctor and his recommendation for surgery, the physician tried to neutralize the situation by joking that he would find the patient a surgeon "who needed the money." By making such a joke the doctor implicitly acknowledged that he knew what the patient really thought of him, yet simultaneously dismissed her opinion as laughable and unserious.

Finally, doctors and staff members often neutralize patients' expressions of watchfulness or mistrust by treating them as "inappropriate behavior." By labeling a patient's alarm as inappropriate doctors not only dismiss the expression of mistrust but may in extreme cases also disqualify the patient from the ranks of persons whose remarks must be taken into account. In most cases the patient is treated in ways that will inhibit any further expressions along these lines.

For example, following cardiac surgery one patient grew accustomed to the regular, even sounds emanating from his cardiac monitor, and these sounds reassured him that his heart was functioning well. When the sounds of his heartbeat suddenly became highly irregular one evening, he became alarmed and rang for the nurse, stating that he felt something was wrong with his heart because the sounds had changed. The nurse briskly replied: "That monitor is none of your business. It's my business, so why don't you just leave it to me."

When staff members respond to indications of mistrust as "inappropriate" they usually apply a wide range of "punishments" to the patient, ranging from gentle rebuke to more extreme measures. An example of the milder response involved a young male patient who was very well liked by the residents and interns. Upon entering his room on rounds one morning, the house officers came upon this patient as he was reading reprints from medical journals about his own particular disease. One of the residents grabbed the reprints from the patient's hands and demanded, "Where did you get these?" "From my brother," replied the patient. The resident continued, "Who's your brother?" The patient smiled and answered, "John." The resident then lectured the patient about how it was "dangerous" for non-medical people to read medical journals because they couldn't understand what they were reading and might reach the wrong conclusions about their illness. After the resident left with the reprints the intern added, "You know, you could have asked us if you had any questions."

From the patient's point of view, the wish to read medical journals (like the tendency to ask questions) might have actually reflected not mistrust of the doctors but rather curiosity and a desire to know more about his illness. Such an interest is often interpreted and treated by doctors, however, as a sign of deficient trust, which is "inappropriate." In making this interpretation they reverse their usual tendency to *underestimate* the patient's mistrust.

When patients attend to what they are supposed to ignore, critical assessments are likely to be made about their characters and personalities. For example, one patient had been kept awake night after night by the sounds of laughter and flirtation between the nurse and orderly who worked on the night shift. The patient had asked her roommate if she would mind if they kept the door to their room closed at night, in order to shut out the noise from the corridor, but her roommate felt she could not sleep with the door closed, since she felt "shut-in." As the laughter one night grew louder and louder, the patient, at three A.M., finally got out of bed, walked to the desk, and asked the nurse and orderly to keep their voices down. That night, the nurse recorded in the patient's chart that the patient "appeared to be nervous and anxious, complained of inability to sleep, and was out of bed walking the corridors." No mention was made of why the patient had been unable to sleep.

Sometimes a complaint or expression of mistrust will be

interpreted by doctors as so "inappropriate" as to justify regarding the patient as mentally disturbed. By labeling a patient
"crazy," doctors ultimately have the power to dismiss any
criticism voiced by a patient. One patient who had been described by the staff as "uncooperative" and a "management
problem" kept a diary in which he logged the comings and
goings of the staff, and the number of minutes it took for
nurses to respond to patient calls. The patient kept the diary
unobtrusively in the night table by his bed, but each time he
was sent to the x-ray department, the residents would remove
the diary from the drawer and laugh together as they read
aloud selected excerpts. The entries in the diary were cited by
the residents as evidence that the patient was "paranoid."
Although the diary seemed peculiar to the residents, it made
perfect sense from the patient's point of view. The patient had
earlier in the week had the unfortunate experience of spending much of one night with a patient-roommate whose death
had gone unnoticed until breakfast time the following morning, an oversight that the patient attributed to the laziness of
the nurses. He had subsequently taken to recording nurse
arrival times in order to demonstrate his argument that the
hospital nursing care was poor.

The doctor's behavior is usually more sympathetic when
patient expressions of mistrust are masked or ambiguous
enough to be handled by indirect responses such as joking or
redefining the situation. A patient who is more direct in
expressing his dissatisfaction is more likely to receive a sharper
reply to his expression of doubts or misgivings. The same
may be said about patient requests for reassurance from doctors (which may themselves be taken as signs of mistrust).
When the requests for reassurance are made indirectly, the
doctor's responses will probably be generous. For example,
when one preoperative patient wished her surgeon "good
luck" in her operation, the doctor responded to the implicit
fear in her communication by reassuring her, saying, "We're
going to do the best we can for you, and everything is working in your favor. When you wake up, the respirator will be

breathing for you, so you won't have to worry about a thing."

On the other hand, when another patient made a more direct demand for reassurance from her surgeon on the night before surgery, asking, "Doctor, will I be all right?" the surgeon curtly replied, "Madam, we don't guarantee our work." And when another preoperative patient shook her head worriedly and remarked: "I hope God is with you tomorrow," the surgeon replied with irritation, "Madam, God has nothing to do with this."

Perhaps with direct requests for reassurance patients call too much attention to the fact that they are entrusting their lives to the doctor, and implicitly charge the doctor with full responsibility for the outcome. Many doctors report feeling uneasy when a patient says, "You're the boss, Doc, whatever you want to do, go ahead." For while the doctor wants full control, he doesn't wish to have the full responsibility dumped in his lap. It is at such moments that physicians often protest (by refusing to "guarantee" the work) that the patient is the one, after all, who "decided" on the operation and must take responsibility for the outcome.

Finally, it must be added that instead of neutralizing indications of patient mistrust, doctors occasionally directly acknowledge and "discuss" the mistrust with the patient. Sometimes these direct confrontations will be made in the hope of arriving at a better relationship with the patient. But more often they are used to threaten the patient with withdrawal from the case, and the result is usually to make the patient less openly critical of the doctor. As one surgeon explained, "Whenever a patient asks me if I mind bringing in a consultant for a second opinion, I say to myself, 'This patient is trouble—this is the kind of patient who is looking for a malpractice suit,' and I tell the patient that if he doesn't fully trust me, he's perfectly welcome to go home and find himself another doctor."

Such a threat of withdrawal is one of the most powerful and effective tactics a doctor can employ to stop or control expressions of patient complaints or mistrust. Most patients, when threatened with physician abandonment at a time when they are extremely vulnerable and helpless, will grimly swallow their concerns and apologize to the doctor, requesting forgiveness for having behaved badly. Frightened by the doctor's anger when they are dependent and see little choice, patients usually figure that the doctor must be retained at all cost. Indeed, many patients fear that if a doctor is angry with them, or dislikes them, he is likely to do a worse job on them, especially in surgery.

This broadly enforced enactment of "trust" has enormous consequences for patient care. By having his thoughts and feelings of doubt and criticism subjected to this complicated neutralization process, the patient becomes easy to control from the staff's point of view. The patient, meanwhile, comes to rely less and less upon his own judgment and observational capacities, since these receive no social validation and may even bring sharp rebuke. And while he may earn some small amount of comfort in being able to ignore frightening information, the patient also loses whatever small amount of autonomy he held in the situation. The ultimate result is to grant complete license to the physician and the staff, a license which is already virtually free from any professional regulation.

In daily life individuals normally monitor their surroundings for signs of danger, since survival ordinarily depends upon continuous watchfulness. The fact that most individuals unhesitatingly entrust their bodies and lives to doctors about whom they know nothing is a remarkable testimony to the power of social conventions and etiquette. For it demonstrates that even our most supposedly spontaneous responses, those involving trust and mistrust, are ultimately felt, not according to "authentic inner" experiences, but rather according to frameworks of social reality and behavioral proprieties that are created and sustained by organizations and institutions.

CONCLUSION

ELIOT FREIDSON, a noted medical sociologist, has pointed out [1] that when physicians assert their right to control the practice of medicine without any interference from the public, they do so on the basis of three claims: first, that medical knowledge is too difficult and esoteric for lay persons to understand; second, that what they do is based upon "objective science"; and third, that as professionals they can be trusted to serve the public's interests rather than their own.

As Freidson carefully argues, however, we must distinguish the specific *knowledge* of the medical profession from decisions about the circumstances and conditions in which that knowledge is to be applied. For while physicians have special expertise in the scientific and technical aspects of medicine, they do not have special expertise in its application. Furthermore, when they control the application of knowledge (as they do now), they inevitably do so in a self-interested rather than public-interested manner, and furthermore, they usurp powers and choices that rightfully belong to the public. In stating this argument, Freidson makes a useful analogy to the case of building new roads:

> . . . we can all agree that how a road is to be built is a technical question best handled by engineers and other experts. But whether a road *should* be built at all, and *where* it should be located are not wholly esoteric technical questions. There are certainly technical considerations which must be taken into account in *evaluating* whether and where a road should be built, but engineering science contains no special expertise to allow it to decide whether a road is "necessary" and what route "must" be taken. Expertise properly plays a major role in suggesting

that already available routes are crowded and determining which routes for a new road would be the easiest and cheapest to construct, but it is social, economic, and political evaluation, not the science of engineering, which, in the light of knowledge, determines whether and where to build a road. Such evaluation is normative in character and is not so esoteric as to justify its restriction to experts. Where laymen are excluded from such evaluation, true expertise is not at issue but rather the social and political power of the expert.[2]

As Freidson elaborates, expertise is often used to mask the power and privilege of the experts rather than to serve the public interest. This is especially true in medicine, where the physician is allowed more influence over public affairs and the practice of applying medical knowledge than his particular expertise genuinely qualifies him for. As Freidson illustrates, although physicians claim to be guided in their work by scientific objectivity, to a large extent what they do depends less upon scientific knowledge than upon moral decisions about how to apply that knowledge. When they decide what should be viewed as sickness, and what treated, and in what manner, and what patients should be told, and what alternatives offered, they are acting not only or even primarily in terms of neutral scientific evidence, but rather from perspectives that inevitably reflect and protect their own positions and interests.

Such biases need not depend upon bad intentions; they follow naturally from the fact that members of every group, physicians included, come to see the world in ways that reflect their particular (and limited) experiences and interests. Thus, given the ambiguity that generally characterizes events, a physician is more likely to diagnose for sickness than for health, and to prescribe a treatment rather than let things take their natural course. And a surgeon is more likely than a medical doctor to suggest (and sincerely believe in) a surgical intervention rather than a medical therapy for a given condition. And, given the choice of waiting and watching or proceeding with surgical intervention in a case of possible appendicitis, it is frequently observed that the surgeon's choice is likely to be seriously affected by the time of the day. For if the patient appears at the hospital with symptoms suggesting appendicitis early in the day, the surgeon may "wait and see" what develops over the next few hours. But if the patient appears with the same symptoms in the early evening, the surgeon is more likely to weigh the balance of the decision in favor of immediate operation, in order to avoid the possibility of being dragged out of bed in the middle of the night and having to come back to the hospital to perform the surgery.

Similarly, it has been widely observed that in geographical areas with a high ratio of surgeons to population, the "indications" for surgery are likely to be interpreted more leniently. Thus medical decisions are based upon more than purely "scientific" considerations; they are based on the convenience, interests and limited perspectives of those who make them.

Many of the incidents and situations described in this book can be seen as illustrations of this basic theme. For example, when staff members of the Emergency Room punish members of the public who arrive with conditions that are not truly "emergencies" (that is, emergencies *as defined by the staff*), what is involved is an application of knowledge involving a group-interested judgment rather than a merely "scientific" response. For, certainly, what is merely routine or unserious to the staff (such as a child who has possibly swallowed a bottle of aspirins) may be experienced as an emergency by the parent. As the sociologist Everett Hughes has pointed out,[3] a common tension in client-professional interactions emerges from the fact that what is an emergency for the client is routine for the professional, and the matter is usually resolved in favor of the professional's perspective.

My analysis of medical mistakes and incompetence indicates how physicians' responses to these events are characterized not by scientific investigation but rather by rationalizations, justifications and emotional demonstrations. And in their tendency to blame patient-victims for medical errors, physicians demonstrate just how far their actual behavior may stray from their claims about being client service-oriented rather than self-interested.

The chapters in this book describing conflicts between the housestaff and private physicians illustrate how physicians' views of illness and proper treatment are not based wholly upon universally shared scientific standards, but rather vary considerably according to the special positions and interests of the particular doctors. Thus, a resident's view of what constitutes an illness deserving of hospitalization is very different from the interpretation of an attending doctor.

Finally, we must consider the claim made by physicians that their knowledge is too complicated and esoteric for lay-persons to understand, and the corollary implications: first, that the public is unable to evaluate the work that physicians do, and second, that patients are unable to take an active, intelligent, indeed, controlling role in decisions about their treatment. I have earlier commented on the importance of distinguishing the technical aspects of medical knowledge from its application, and the point that the application depends upon moral judgments that can only be properly made by the public. But what about the patient who is deemed incapable of making decisions in his own behalf? As Freidson points out, there will certainly be occasional patients who are too ignorant or upset to participate effectively in decisions about their own treatment, but doctors unjustifiably ascribe these incapacities to *all* patients in order to maximize their own autonomy and interests:

> Indeed, the customary professional characterization of the client . . . insists on his ignorance and irrationality. Such characterization is the prime justification for the profession's inclination to make the client at best a passive participant in the work—to, in essence, remove from the client his everyday status as an adult citizen, to minimize his essential capacity to reason and his right to dignity. Expertise in general claims its privilege by claiming the client's incapacity.[4]

Moreover, Freidson's evaluation of the "information" which is given to patients comes very close to my own observations:

In spite of recent federal requirements that clients participating as "subjects" in research give "informed consent," and in spite of the legal releases required for such procedures as surgery, it is my impression that clients are more often bullied than informed into consent, their resistance weakened in part by their desire for the general service if not the specific procedure, in part by the oppressive setting they find themselves in, and in part by the calculated intimidation, restriction of information, and covert threats of rejection by the professional staff itself.[5]

We arrive, finally, at the question of how we are to bring health care under more effective evaluation and regulation to assure that patients' interests are truly served. Until recently, physicians have gone unchallenged in their claim to be the best and only source of critical review. Such a privilege has been part of their overall autonomy. Pressured only recently by threats of government and institutional intervention (which I shall discuss below) doctors have stridently argued that meaningful regulation can come only from within their own ranks. Now, doctors have proposed that formal and informal "peer-review" should take place at local levels, through such mechanisms as I have described in this book: mortality and morbidity review conferences, departmental supervision and utilization review committees. In fact, utilization review is now a federal requirement for qualifying for Medicare and Medicaid payments and is known as Physicians' Service Review Organizations (PSRO's). My description and analysis of some of these peer-review mechanisms indicate how ineffective I believe them to be. Eliot Freidson draws the same conclusion:

> So long as the profession places heavy reliance on criteria established by personal or clinical experience and judgment, so long as it emphasizes good intentions rather than good performance, and so long as its characteristic disciplinary device is a form of exclusion which operates to segregate levels of performance into relatively homogeneous groups of practitioners, each group with different clinical prejudices, the profession cannot really regulate itself.[6]

Clarification is needed on one point that Freidson raises,

in light of my own research. Freidson suggests that the primary disciplinary action taken against incompetent or unethical physicians is to exclude them from the staff of a particular hospital or organization and thereby further isolate them from needed assistance and supervision, while still allowing them to practice on unsuspecting patients. Although this may indeed be the primary form of discipline, I have nonetheless personally found such actions to be very rare. Indeed, some of the department chiefs I described explicitly named the problem Freidson raises as their reason for allowing incompetent physicians to retain hospital privileges. Whatever the actual frequency of such suspensions, it is obvious that disciplinary action rarely goes any further, and I am sure that for other reasons the process of segregating levels of performance which Freidson describes does take place in a widespread, systematic manner. For doctors are ranked, relatively early in their training (indeed, on the basis of where they went to medical school and did their residencies), into "classes" with differential prestige and opportunities, and doctors are likely to travel within these rankings for the rest of their careers.

The most important point is that neither keeping incompetent doctors on a hospital staff nor releasing them to less prestigious organizations is a satisfactory solution to the problems of medical regulation. For certainly patients are never informed of critical peer evaluations and certainly doctors are extremely reluctant to pass judgment on each other's work. Furthermore, the problem of "incompetent" doctors is only a small part of the difficulty, since physicians allow even competent members of their ranks to engage routinely in questionable activities, given the fact that medical choices are based upon self-interested perspectives. At this juncture, it is necessary to step back to take a look at the broader political, economic and social changes currently appearing in the American health care system which will play important roles in matters of regulation and quality of care.

Up until now we have exclusively examined physicians as

the major or dominant group controlling health care policies and the application of medical knowledge. But increasingly, the power of doctors is being challenged by another important group. This second group is *not* consumers, for the public does not presently constitute any significant threat to those who are in control. Robert Alford, a sociologist who has written about the politics of health care, has described [7] this second group as composed of individuals who direct large organizations and empires in the health system. They include directors of insurance companies, hospital administrators, medical school directors and public health officials. As Alford explains, the traditionally dominant group (the practicing and research physicians) wish to maintain professional autonomy in their work, competition among practitioners and services, and physician control over hospitals, medical schools and public health agencies. In contrast, the challenging group of institutional directors wishes to extend control of their organizations over the work lives of physicians and other employees in the health system (thereby reducing the status of physicians to merely another group of salaried employees). Their aim is to extend public financing and to coordinate and centralize health services through organizations such as Health Maintenance Organizations (HMO's). Their goal is to use more efficiently the expensive technology which they expect will be increasingly central to health care.

It has been pointed out that such a challenge to the autonomy of physicians has become possible as a result of the decline of solo practice among physicians.[8] Because of the increasing importance of science and high technology in American medicine, physicians have become increasingly reliant on hospitals and other organizations in their work, and increasingly unable to privately control their fee-for-service practices. As one analyst predicts, our medical care system eventually will probably be

> financed through Federal tax revenues, dominated by private insurance companies operating through HMO's and reducing the medical profession to a group of hired professional en-

gineers. Within ten years we shall be marketing medical care the same way we are now marketing automobiles—and with similar hazards.[9]

Doctors' own recognition that they are becoming "mere employees" of large organizations is of course consistent with the widespread appearance, for the first time in American history, of doctors' strikes. But although there is at first an attractive ring to the demands of the challenging group for better planning and efficiency in health care, a closer look suggests that since large profits are involved, certain segments of this group will try to cut the costs ultimately in order to maximize the profits for the huge corporations that will dominate the American health care system: multinational corporations involved in insurance, finance, pharmaceutical, electronics, and medical supply industries. Of course, this challenging group is composed of diverse members with very different purposes, and many individuals may be advocating programs that they sincerely feel will improve medical care with no personal gain for themselves. And there may even be some short-term apparent benefits to health care in these programs. Nonetheless, the overall thrust of this movement will probably move in ways that maximize profits for private industries rather than maximize benefits for consumers.

Indeed, as the annual expenditures on health care jumped from 26 billion dollars in 1960 to 67 billion dollars in 1970, to over 94 billion dollars in 1973, and almost 120 billion in 1975,[10] the giant corporations that dominate other areas of American life have diversified into health care, and they are enjoying huge profits.[11] It has been reported, for example, that from 1970 to 1973 the profits of the private health-insurance industry increased by a record 120%.[12] And pharmaceutical and medical supply industries have also profited handsomely in recent years.[13] These profits are paid for by the public, not only through the rising costs of medical care and insurance, but also because federal income taxes are paying for an ever-increasing proportion of health care costs. As one sociologist described it:

> . . . the word *profit* is critical here. It must be kept in mind
> that a great deal of money can be made in the health field . . .
> because of the relationships between hospitals, physicians, sup-
> pliers, and the Federal government, ordinary "market" rules are
> not as operative here. . . . As in the military-industrial com-
> plex, market mechanisms are altered by the members of the
> complex to their advantage—and to the ultimate disadvantage
> of the consumers who pay the final bill.[14]

We have earlier seen the problems of "peer-review" regulation of medical practice by physicians. What kind of regulation of health care can we expect in this shift away from
physician-practitioner dominance to corporate control? Others
have pointed to a considerable overlap between the corporate
domination in the health industries and the corporate domination in other spheres of the American economy, as well as
an overlap between corporations, research-funding institutions and the executive and legislative branches of the federal
government that oversee and "regulate" the activities of the
health care system.[15] Certainly we can expect that with the
strong influence of medical supply and electronics industries,
there will be a push toward expensive, high-technology therapies and medical equipment, frequently of doubtful benefit
to patients. Certainly we can expect that with the powerful
influence of the insurance companies and their concern with
profits, attempts will be made to cut the costs of medical care
in ways that may also cut the quality of that care. For when
large profits are involved in health care policies, those who
dominate the industry and policymaking bodies will organize
health care for their own gain.

In considering a few of the political and economic forces
at play in health care, I have wandered considerably from
my original focus—staff behavior in a hospital—but such an
excursion is necessary for two reasons. One is that in examining the ways that physicians have failed to regulate health
care practices to best serve the interests of the consumers, it
should not be assumed that the new planners and managers of
health care will serve the public's interests any better. Just as

physicians have regulated medical practice to maximize their autonomy and profits, so will the giant corporations and their administrators use the health industry to build up power and profits. And many planners working in this direction may be unaware of the ultimate consequences of this trend, and, like physicians, unaware of how their apparently "objective" calculations follow from the perspectives of those who stand to gain from these policies.

Just as physicians have "regulated" medical practice in ways consistent with their own interests, so will the giant corporations and their administrators do the same. Just because this book has focused upon the problems of physician behavior and physician-consumer conflicts of interest, I would not want the reader to wrongly conclude that these are the only reasons for the poor treatment and large bills patients receive. New, expensive medical innovations of doubtful value to patients are already being produced by the large corporations that are coming to dominate American health care. What comes next may be worse than what we have known before.

The second reason for introducing this broader perspective in the conclusion is that it provides a background for understanding some of the conflicts and developments in "Lakeside" hospital. For the patterns that exist in the broad economic and political spheres of American life and health care are reproduced on the smaller local levels of individual hospitals. As the reader will recall, the private attending physicians described in this book were forever in conflict with the "organization" of the hospital, represented by its chiefs, administrators and housestaff. What was at stake for them was not only profits but also autonomy and control over the conditions of their work. The conflicts I have described in the daily life of the hospital, then, significantly reflect the competing interest groups and the play of forces at work in the larger society.

The kind of analysis this book offers does not lend itself to simple suggestions for improving medical care. I hope I have made the reader more informed about some aspects of hospital life that would not otherwise be obvious. Perhaps this information will be useful to individuals who wish to resist the passive and helpless positions into which patients are pushed, as well as assist the public in evaluating and influencing developments in medical practice and health-care policy.

As for the larger problem, I am convinced that as long as medical care and its practice are organized to provide profits, convenience and power to special-interest groups—whether they be physicians or the owners and directors of large organizations and corporations—the interests of most of the public will not be protected. Our health care system will not truly serve the needs and welfare of the public until it is separated from profitmaking enterprises.

NOTES

1. Eliot Freidson, *The Profession of Medicine* (New York: Dodd, Mead and Co., 1970). Especially chapters 15 and 16.
2. Freidson, p. 336.
3. Everett Hughes, "Mistakes At Work," *The Sociological Eye: Book 2, Work, Self and the Study of Society* (Chicago: Aldine, 1970), p. 316.
4. Freidson, p. 353.
5. Freidson, p. 376.
6. Freidson, pp. 366–367.
7. Robert Alford, "The Political Economy of Health Care: Dynamics Without Change," *Politics and Society* (1972), vol. 2: 127–164. Also, *Health Care Politics: Ideological and Interest Group Barriers to Reform* (Chicago: University of Chicago Press, 1975).
8. Several writers have made this point. For a clear description of this historical trend, see Sander Kelman, "Toward the Political Economy of Medical Care," *Inquiry,* vol. 8, no. 3 (1971), pp. 30–38.
9. Kelman, p. 35.
10. Alford, 1972; and W. W. Scott, "Professional Freedom and Governmental Control," *Annals of Surgery,* vol. 180, no. 4 (1974), p. 180. Also *San Francisco Chronicle,* April 26, 1976, p. 1.
11. See, for example, Howard Waitzkin and Barbara Waterman, *The Exploitation of Illness in Capitalist Society* (Indianapolis: Bobbs-Merrill, 1974), and Vicente Navarro, "Social Policy Issues: An Explanation of the Composition, Nature, and Func-

tions of the Present Health Sector of the United States," *Bulletin of the New York Academy of Medicine,* vol. 51, no. 1 (January 1975), pp. 199–234.
12. Navarro, 1975, p. 228.
13. Waitzkin and Waterman, p. 12.
14. Elliott Krause, "Health and the Politics of Technology," *Inquiry,* vol. 8, no. 3 (1971), pp. 51–59.
15. Vicente Navarro, "The Industrialization of Fetishism or The Fetishism of Industrialization: A Critique of Ivan Illich," *International Journal of Health Services,* vol. 5, no. 3 (1976), pp. 363–364.

SUGGESTIONS FOR READING

MY PERSPECTIVES ON HOSPITAL LIFE and on American health care have been shaped not only by my own research observations, but also by the work of other sociologists. I would like to review these influences and suggest some additional reading for those who would like to delve further into the subject.

My overall theoretical and substantive orientation in studying social behavior has been influenced most directly by the work of Erving Goffman. I enthusiastically recommend any of Goffman's books to the reader, especially the following: *Asylums: Essays on the Social Situation of Mental Patients and Other Inmates* (Garden City: Doubleday Anchor, 1961); *Interaction Ritual: Essays on Face-to-Face Behavior* (Garden City: Doubleday Anchor, 1967); *Stigma: Notes on the Management of Spoiled Identity* (Englewood Cliffs: Prentice-Hall, 1963; *Encounters* (Indianapolis: Bobbs-Merrill Co., Inc., 1961); *Strategic Interaction* (Philadelphia: University of Pennsylvania Press, 1969); *Relations In Public* (New York: Harper and Row, 1971); *Frame Analysis* (Cambridge: Harvard University Press, 1974). Readers interested in hospital life should probably read *Asylums* first, for it is a brilliant study of staff and patient life in a mental hospital, with extraordinary applicability to other institutional settings.

Another important influence on my orientation is a collection of essays by Everett C. Hughes, *The Sociological Eye: Book 2, Work, Self and the Study of Society* (Chicago: Aldine, 1970). Many of my ideas about medical mistakes and about client-practitioner relations are drawn from Hughes' essay, "Mistakes at Work," and several essays on the professions which appear in that collection.

An excellent and comprehensive analysis of the organization and perspectives of physicians can be found in Eliot Freidson's *The Profession of Medicine* (New York: Dodd, Mead and Co., 1970). I also recommend Freidson's other books, *Professional Dominance,* (New York: Atherton, 1970), and *Medical Men and their Work: A Sociological Reader* (co-edited with Judith Lorber) (Chicago: Aldine, 1972). Freidson's most recent book is about "peer-review," *Doctoring Together: A Study of Professional Self-Control* (New York: Elsevier, 1976). For an introduction to some of the implications of the spreading power of medical institutions in this society, I recommend Irving Zola, "Medicine as an Institution of Social Control," *Sociological Review,* 20: 4 (November, 1972).

Those who would like to read about the training and socialization of physicians should look at Howard Becker, et al., *Boys in White: Student Culture in Medical School* (Chicago: University of Chicago Press, 1961). An excellent study of families' experiences with illness and with hospitals is Fred Davis, *Passage Through Crisis: Polio Victims and their Families* (Indianapolis: Bobbs-Merrill, 1963). Another interesting study of hospital life from the patient's perspective is Julius A. Roth, *Timetables: Structuring the Passage of Time in Hospital Treatment and Other Careers* (Indianapolis: Bobbs-Merrill, 1963). A very thoughtful essay about how medical diagnoses and treatment may reflect institutional concerns rather than "objective" symptoms is Arlene Kaplan Daniels, "The Social Construction of Military Psychiatric Diagnoses," in Hans Peter Dreitzel, ed., *Recent Sociology, No. 2* (New York: Macmillan, 1970). There have been several excellent books about the sociology of dying in medical institutions, most notably David Sudnow, *Passing On* (Englewood Cliffs: Prentice-Hall, 1967), and two studies by Barney Glaser and Anselm Strauss, *Awareness of Dying* (Chicago: Aldine, 1965) and *Time For Dying* (Chicago: Aldine, 1968).

My chapter on the enactment of trust was influenced by the work of others who have examined how social reality is "negotiated" in ongoing interactions. One of the important theoretical treatments of this subject is P. Berger and T. Luckman, *The Social Construction of Reality* (New York: Doubleday Anchor, 1967). My essay on trust was more directly influenced by two essays by Joan Emerson, especially, "Behavior In Private Places: Sustaining Definitions of Reality in Gynecological Examinations," in Hans Peter Dreitzel, ed., *Recent Sociology, No. 2* (New York: Macmillan, 1970); and also her essay, "Nothing Unusual Is Happening," in T. Shibutani ed., *Human Nature and Collective Behavior* (Englewood Cliffs: Prentice-Hall, 1970). My thoughts about trust were also stimulated by Erving Goffman's reflections about stealing, concealing and revealing information in his essay, "Expression Games" in *Strategic Interaction,* his essay "Normal Appearances" in *Relations in Public,* and his book *Frame Analysis,* all cited above.

For those who would like to read about the political and economic factors shaping health care policy, I highly recommend an article by Robert Alford, "The Political Economy of Health Care: Dynamics Without Change," in *Politics and Society* 2: 127–164 (1972), and also Alford's recent book, *Health Care Politics: Ideological and Interest Group Barriers To Reform* (Chicago: University of Chicago Press, 1975). Other very useful books on this subject include Howard B. Waitzkin and Barbara Waterman, *The Exploitation of Illness in Capitalist Society* (Indianapolis: Bobbs-Merrill, 1974), and Barbara and John Ehrenreich, *The American Health Empire: Power, Profit and Politics* (New York: Vintage, 1971). Several excellent articles have appeared in the last few years which outline a framework for viewing American health care in political, economic and historical terms. Among them is an essay by Sander Kelman, "Toward the Political Economy of Medical Care," *Inquiry,* 1971, vol. 8, no. 3, and in the same journal issue, an article by Elliott Krause, "Health Care and the Politics of Technology." Also highly recommended are several essays by Vicente Navarro including, "Social Policy Issues: An Explanation of the Composition, Nature, and Functions of the Present Health Sector of the United States," in *Bulletin of the New York Academy of Medicine,* vol. 51, no. 1 (January, 1975); and also, "The Industrialization of Fetishism or the Fetishism of Industrialization: A Critique of Ivan Illich," in the *International Journal of Health Services,* vol. 5, no. 3 (1975).

Finally, there are several interesting essays about the advantages, problems and complexities of doing sociological field work. Among these I recommend Kai Erickson, "A Comment on Disguised Observation in Sociology," in *Social Problems,* vol. 14, no. 4, reprinted in William J. Filstead, ed., *Qualitative Methodology* (Chicago: Markham, 1970). Also recommended is Howard Becker and Blanche Geer, "Participant Observation and Interviewing: A Comparison," *Human Organization,* vol. 16 (1957), pp. 28–32 (and also reprinted in Filstead, cited above). Another useful book is by Rosalie Wax, *Doing Fieldwork: Warnings and Advice* (Chicago: University of Chicago Press, 1974). And finally, for one of the most insightful and entertaining essays about doing participant-observation research, the reader should see Arlene Kaplan Daniels, "The Low-Caste Stranger in Social Research," in Gideon Sjoberg, ed., *Politics, Ethics and Social Research* (Cambridge: Schenkman, 1967).

APPENDIX

CORONARY ARTERY BYPASS SURGERY: LAISSEZ-FAIRE IN AMERICAN SURGICAL EXPERIMENTS

INTRODUCTION

In the appendix that follows, I present a case history of a surgical innovation that is sweeping the nation's hospitals. But despite its popularity, coronary artery bypass surgery can be shown to carry significant risks, very limited benefits, and enormous public expense. Furthermore, the operation developed in a destructively unregulated manner and has been adopted for wide use before the demonstration of its long-term value, either for individual patients or for the public as a whole. It is routinely performed by inexperienced surgeons in badly equipped hospitals. And yet, the American public believes it to be a miracle of modern medicine.

I chose to include this appendix for several reasons. First, a large number of people are consenting to have the surgery with very mistaken ideas of how it may help them and how it may hurt them. Second, a detailed look at this surgery provides another opportunity to observe how medical practice in the United States may be shaped more by economic, professional and political considerations than by "scientific" evidence or concern with the welfare of patients and the public. Third, the history of this operation illustrates the total absence of any institutions or regulatory mechanisms for protecting public welfare in the development and practice of new surgical practices. Finally, the operation exemplifies many disturbing trends in contemporary health care.

By shifting our attention away from life within a hospital to the history of a surgical innovation, we change our vantage point. But in doing so we may have another, broader look at the same issues we have considered throughout the book.

CORONARY ARTERY BYPASS SURGERY: LAISSEZ-FAIRE IN AMERICAN SURGICAL EXPERIMENTS

CORONARY ARTERY BYPASS surgery may be the most momentous innovation in contemporary American medicine. Some analysts have predicted on the basis of present trends that in ten years this operation could be a 100 billion dollar a year industry; it could dominate not only our health budget but a large part of our national resources.[1,2] The operation has already become one of the most widely used and costly medical procedures performed in the United States. In 1976, close to 80,000 patients in over five hundred hospitals will undergo open heart surgery for "repair" of their coronary arteries, with an average bill of about $12,000 per patient. Hundreds more local community hospitals are tooling up to do the operation, with an expectation that there will be a greater and greater patient demand. When all the hidden costs of the operation are considered, it appears that in 1976 close to three billion dollars will be spent on coronary bypass surgery.

What is coronary artery bypass surgery? (Its full name is saphenous vein coronary artery surgery.) It is a procedure in which the occluded portions of the three major coronary arteries carrying blood to the heart are bypassed with the insertion of grafts made from a vein taken from the patient's leg. The idea behind the operation is to surgically create new pathways around the occluded portions of the coronary arteries (by inserting bypass grafts between the aorta and the arteries, past the points of occlusion) in order to bring an increased flow of blood to the heart.

Since the procedure was first done in its modern form eight

years ago, the goals of the operation have remained the same. They are threefold: 1) to relieve chest pain (angina pectoris) caused by insufficient oxygen supply to the heart and to enable the individual to tolerate more activity and exercise; 2) to prevent heart attacks and the deterioration of the heart muscle; 3) to prolong life.

The surgery has had an enormously enthusiastic response from surgeons and patients. Much of the enthusiasm has come from the operation's dramatic success in treating chest pain: the surgery eliminates or relieves angina pectoris in 75 to 85 percent or more of the cases.

Patients who are relieved of chest pain often assume that they have been miraculously "cured" of their heart disease. But they are wrong. In fact, the operation is merely a temporary palliative measure that treats symptoms for a limited period of time. The surgery is *not* a cure for coronary artery disease, which is a chronic, progressive disease. It has not yet been demonstrated that the operation either prolongs life or prevents heart attacks. Although these claims have been made by some enthusiastic surgeons, this operation has been the source of a great deal of controversy in the medical profession, for there are conflicting views of the benefits of the surgery beyond symptom relief, and there is clear evidence that the *operation itself may cause significant damage to the heart, contains many long-term risks, and actually accelerates the progression of coronary artery disease.*

Despite the controversy and the many unknown facts about the surgery it is clear that the operation is being performed at a startlingly increasing rate. Cardiac surgery facilities and teams are proliferating so quickly that despite the popularity of the operation, hundreds of facilities are significantly underused. This creates a situation of hazard for patients because of inexperienced medical staffs and results in wasteful and unnecessary programs which are paid for by the public. Regardless of these facts, many more hospitals are investing in cardiac surgery programs, creating the likelihood that the operation will be applied on an increasingly broad scale, even before the full facts about the surgery and its benefits and dangers are understood.

As I shall illustrate later, there are many reasons for the wild proliferation of this operation. What seems like senseless or questionable behavior from the point of view of scientific or medical evidence may be explained when the operation is viewed in a larger political, economic, and social context. Some of the reasons for the spread of coronary bypass surgery have to do with the financial interests of those who profit from it: cardiac surgeons who needed to find new sources for operations after their old ones began to disappear and hospitals that overexpanded way beyond market demand and are competing with one another for patients and doctors. Profits also go to medical supply industries and giant electronics firms that diversified into the health industry. Hospitals are providing a needed market for equipment produced by the electronics corporations; indeed, most of the monitoring equipment used in heart surgery was developed in the aerospace program.

In addition to these underlying economic factors, there is a practically limitless number of persons who can be persuaded to have the operation, making it a profitable frontier for those making a financial or career investment in heart surgery. Coronary artery disease affects a huge portion of the population. It is the greatest single cause of death in the United States, and is responsible for a large portion of early death and disability. It has been estimated [3] that at least one third of the males in the U.S. over the age of 55 have significant coronary artery disease. Autopsies conducted on soldiers in Vietnam suggest that the vast majority of even young men already show signs of atherosclerotic disease. The illness is especially prevalent in the segment of the population that controls our national economic and political resources: affluent white males over the age of 45. The media has called a great deal of attention to coronary artery disease and heart attacks, and has created considerable anxiety about the illness, as well as dramatized the miraculous benefits of surgery. Finally, the special nature of the disease, involving severe and anxiety-provoking pain, orients patients to an "activist" approach and readiness for surgical intervention. All of these factors create the conditions for a wide demand for the operation, especially since the public has an erroneous view of its benefits and hazards. As some physicians have remarked, many patients do not even consult with their family physicians. They make their own diagnoses and go straight to a cardiac surgeon. And now many hospitals and physicians have taken an "activist" approach to seeking out a broad range of patients, including those in an early stage of the disease who are advised to undergo the operation "prophylactically."

Coronary bypass surgery has been very successful in relieving chest pain and increasing exercise tolerance, and there is some evidence that it may also prolong life and prevent heart attacks in *selected* subgroups of patients. But present evidence indicates that these subgroups make up only a *small percentage* of all those patients suffering from angina who undergo the operation. Despite these surgical benefits, when one considers the present and past facts about the operation, and their broader implications, there is reason to be alarmed about its rapid proliferation on three grounds:

1) First, there is a great discrepancy between what patients believe about the operation's efficacy and what has actually been scientifically demonstrated. Many patients have erroneous ideas about both the risks and the benefits of the surgery; they are misled both by doctors and the media.

2) The operation has been developed and applied in a completely unregulated fashion: often to the detriment of the patients undergoing the procedure. There are no restrictions in this country about the introduction and application of experimental surgical procedures. There are no specifications about who may do them or for what reason. There is no requirement that information about their performance and outcomes be reported in any systematic way. This pervasive lack of regulation has led to inferior care in many cases and the wide clinical application of untested and poorly understood surgical interventions, with a sacrifice of many patients.

3) Coronary bypass surgery illustrates several trends in American health care that must be critically examined. As this operation comes to dominate our health resources it is paid for by the American public (not just by those who have the operation) either directly by federal taxes that subsidize the purchase of equipment or by increased health and insurance costs. Unnecessary expansion of cardiac surgery facilities creates not only poor care but expenses that are passed on to the public. Much of this money eventually winds up as profits for large corporations involved in the health industry.

Coronary artery surgery is part of a larger trend in which American medicine is increasingly dominated by expensive, high-technology diagnostic procedures and treatments. The benefits for patients of this medical technology are doubtful in many instances, yet there has been an unquestioned tendency on the part of the public and physicians to assume that the technology is useful, justified, and soundly applied. Lately the media has been calling attention to certain "moral" or "ethical" problems introduced by the expansion of technology in medicine (for example, questions like "when do you pull the plug"), but little attention has been given to a broader analysis of the role of technology in medicine and questions such as the "ethicality" and impact of huge corporate profits in our health care system.[4] Given the expansion of expensive technology in medicine, the idea of what is "necessary" and what is "unnecessary" surgery must now require a consideration of what is good for society as a whole as well as what is good for individual recipients.

I—THE FACTS ABOUT CORONARY ARTERY SURGERY

Most doctors now agree that coronary artery surgery can improve or relieve chest pain in 75–85 percent of the cases. Many studies show that when patients undergoing surgery are compared with those who are medically treated, the ones having surgery experience less pain and are less restricted in activity than those who do not have surgery.[5, 6, 7] Some medical doctors have argued, however, that with very active medical therapy, angina can be relieved in 65–95 percent of the cases *without* surgical intervention.[6]

The benefits of the operation beyond the relief of angina and increased tolerance for exercise have been the source of much disagreement among physicians. As many have pointed out, the relief of symptoms should not be confused with actual physical improvement, and in some cases the relief of symptoms is actually caused by a *worsening* of physical status; in some cases relief of angina is the result of surgery-induced death of heart muscle no longer in pain from inadequate oxygen supply. There have been numerous situations in which patients report relief from pain after surgery which could not objectively have done them any good. Studies have shown that patients reported relief from chest pain after "sham" operations (in which the patient unknowingly underwent only a chest incision and no actual surgery of the coronary vessels) or in cases where vein grafts have become occluded and could not possibly provide increased blood flow to the heart.[8, 9] Thus some of the relief of chest pain after surgery can be attributed to a "placebo" effect and some of it caused by actual damage to the heart muscle. For one of the large risks of the surgery is a heart attack (myocardial infarction), which frequently occurs either during or after the operation. When this happens, pain disappears because heart muscle previously alive but in need of more oxygen (creating pain) becomes dead, scarred, and no longer painful.[10]

Recently many surgeons have claimed on the basis of their "trial runs" that the operation *does* produce benefits beyond relief of pain. They claim the surgery increases the chances of survival for those patients suffering from severe disease of multiple vessels (two or three coronary arteries) and especially those suffering from disease of the left main coronary artery. Since these patients ordinarily face a very high risk of having a heart attack, it is argued that surgery to bypass the occlusions is likely to help them live longer and avoid heart attacks. Since the mortality rates of the operation have been brought to a low figure in some medical centers, many surgeons take an active approach to finding patients with occlusions in multiple vessels.[2,5,11]

Indeed, many surgeons, convinced that the operation has benefits beyond relief of symptoms, are operating on patients who do *not* have chest pain (asymptomatic) or who have mild chest pain. Convinced of its power to prolong life, large numbers of surgeons are using the operation as a prophylactic measure against heart attacks. And patients are by and large consenting to the surgery under the impression that the surgery will save their lives.

The widespread use of bypass surgery on the grounds of benefits other than symptom relief has received considerable criticism from many physicians who point out that there has not yet been evidence in controlled studies of increased survival or lowered risk of heart attack as a result of surgery.[6,12,13] As many physicians have noted, surgical reports showing better survival rates for surgically treated patients are often biased and misleading because they involve patient selections biased in favor of good surgical results. They are also misleading because they compare surgical results with *old* data about medical treatments that have now allegedly been considerably improved with the use of recently approved drugs such as Propanolol. Furthermore, it is argued that surgical reports on the benefits of the operation are likely to represent only the best results from the most successful medical centers because the reports are voluntary.[6,14,15,16]

In fact, claims that the operation prolongs life have *not* been confirmed by controlled studies randomly assigning patients to surgical and medical treatment. Only *one* small subgroup of very high-risk patients with chest pain have been shown[13] thus far to benefit from the operation in terms of survival two years after the diagnosis. These are patients who suffer from occlusion of the left main coronary artery, and they comprise about 10 percent of all patients experiencing angina and thus only a small percentage of patients actually having the operation. It would therefore appear on the basis of existing research findings that the vast majority of patients undergoing the operation (about 80 percent) can at this time expect no benefit from the operation other than relief of chest pain and increased tolerance of exercise and activity. Indeed, an official surgical committee composing guidelines for planning and evaluation of cardiac surgery pointed out that although many hospitals are expanding programs on the basis of the surgery's success in relieving pain, "conclusions on long-term benefits with reference to the prevention of infarction [heart attack] and survival await further reports." [17]

Many surgeons have argued that although all of the facts about the operation are not yet known, since it seems to relieve chest pain so well and seems to hold some promise in saving lives and is relatively "safe," it is reasonable to perform the surgery on large numbers of people. But although the mortality rates have been kept low at some medical centers, a closer examination of the operation reveals a large number of serious hazards and problems. These include highly variable risks of mortality and morbidity at the time of surgery, accelerated deterioration of the arteries being bypassed, a high rate of graft occlusions (which lead to heart attacks when combined with the accelerated decline of the arteries) and the reappearance after a few years of severe chest pains because of the progressive nature of the disease, possibly accelerated by the surgery.

Mortality rates (death during surgery or soon afterward) for the operation are generally reported in the range from 2 to 12 percent.[5,6,14,18,19,20,21] A few centers have reported much lower mortality rates than are typical (as low as 1.2 percent),[11] but there is considerable evidence that the more characteristic mortality risk is much higher. One survey of hospital mortality rates with the operation (excluding the one atypical center with unusually low rates) suggested a characteristic mortality incidence of 7.2–11.8 percent.[21] It is also very clear that surgical mortality is related to the experience of the surgeon and the staff. For example, one analysis of the range of mortality rates showed that in surgical reports involving 100 or fewer operations, the overall mortality rate was 12 percent; in reports of 100–200 cases the rate was 9 percent and for reports of 200 or more cases, there was an average mortality of 4.5 percent.[5,14] While it can be argued that as surgeons become more experienced with this procedure the mortality rates will approach the lower figure, it is also unfortunately true that as more and more surgeons offer the operation at typically underused local community facilities, there will be greater numbers of inexperienced teams doing the operation with high mortality outcomes.

Reports of myocardial infarction (heart attack) during surgery also vary considerably. Reports suggest that 5–40 percent [22] of patients undergoing operation experience a heart attack during or soon after surgery. Many suggest that the typical rate of infarction is about 15–25 percent.[6,12,20,23,24] Since one of the arguments in favor of the operation is the prevention of heart attacks, this high incidence of surgery-related infarction must be considered in the evaluation of the surgery. As in the case of mortality rates, the likelihood of this surgical complication seems to be related to the experience of the surgeon [22] as well as the condition of the patient.

Another important consideration in the operation is the "patency rates" or the extent to which the vein bypass grafts stay open or become occluded. There is a tendency for the walls of the vein grafts to become thickened and occluded because they are subjected to arterial pressure. Reports indicate that *20–30 percent of vein grafts become occluded within one year of surgery*,[10,25,26,27] and that patency failures occur more frequently in smaller and less experienced centers.[22,25] Obviously, patients whose grafts become occluded will experience no benefit from the surgery. Long-term experiences with vein grafts in the legs also suggest increased occlusion as time goes by.[6]

The full danger of this tendency for grafts to occlude can only be fully appreciated in the larger context of what the grafting does to the original arteries and their openings. There is now much evidence that the insertion of vein grafts causes significant acceleration of disease in the arteries receiving the grafts. *The insertion of grafts increases the likelihood that new total occlusions will develop in the arteries at points both before and after the graft insertion site.*[22] For example, one major study reported [10] that *just six months after surgery, increased occlusion was found in the arteries of 50 out of 71 patients studied.* New *total* occlusions were found in 30 percent of the 188 major coronary arteries studied. These occlusions developed at different rates according to whether or not a patent (non-occluded) bypass graft was present. New total occlusions developed in only 16 percent of arteries *not* bypassed, in 29 percent of arteries with a patent (open) graft, and in 62 percent of arteries with an occluded graft. This report and others suggest that not only do bypass grafts accelerate the progression of disease in the arteries, but also that one of the dangers of the operation is that when grafts are open early after surgery they encourage a complete obstruction of whatever opening existed in the artery prior to surgery. This is partly because there is less flow of blood going through the artery and the stasis causes occlusion. As long as the grafts are patent, the closure of the arteries is not a problem, but when the grafts themselves become occluded later on (and there is a progressive tendency for this to happen) the patient is in a worse situation than before surgery because he has lost whatever arterial opening he had before and now faces a greater risk of heart attack. As one study suggested,[10] the relief of pain after surgery may in some cases be the result of this surgery-induced arterial obstruction which has resulted in dead heart muscle.

Another problem with the operation is that early hopes that surgery would improve the functioning of the heart muscle have not been substantiated. Researchers have found that bypass grafting has little or no beneficial effect on cardiac function, especially in patients who have had a prior heart attack.[27] Of course, relief from pain and increased tolerance for exercise may still take place even though there is no improvement in the pumping abilities of the left ventricle of the heart.[25] Still other problems may be added to this list: for example, the operation entails risks of phlebitis and infection.

Finally, one of the most discouraging facts about the operation just now becoming evident but hardly a surprise is that the benefits of the surgery substantially decline after a few years. Because of the progressive (possibly accelerated by surgery) nature of atherosclerosis, chest pains eventually begin to reappear in those who have undergone operation. One major study (involving 350 patients) [18] reported that 40 percent of patients experienced a deterioration with respect to chest pain 30 months after surgery, compared to how they felt nine months after surgery (47 percent were unchanged and 13 percent felt better). Such a decline in symptomatic relief can naturally be expected to progress with additional time. The researchers therefore concluded that the initial symptomatic benefits of the operation are not maintained in late follow-up studies, because of the nature of the underlying disease. Thus, the only clearly established benefit of the operation, relief of chest pain, is only a temporary one which declines after a few years. This experience and the logic of the deterioration has been reported in other long-term evaluations of the operation.[22]

Given this information, what do doctors advise their patients? There are several surgical centers specializing in this procedure that argue the operation should be done on a wider rather than a more restricted basis. Since some surgeons have "faith" in the benefits of the operation beyond relief of pain they advocate performing the surgery as a prophylactic measure against heart attacks, and even on patients who do not have chest pain. Physicians with this orientation advocate doing diagnostic tests on patients in no discomfort but who have shown irregularities on electrocardiogram readings. If x-rays reveal narrowing in the coronary arteries of these asymptomatic patients (and this is likely, given the incidence of coronary disease) they advocate surgery. According to many observers, some of these centers, therefore, may accept patients for surgery who are "healthier" than those coming to surgery in other institutions, with a consequent lower mortality rate. This low mortality rate, in turn, earns them more surgical referrals from physicians who are unaware that the good statistics may be partly explained by the selection of patients.

On the other side are the physicians (sometimes called "doves" by surgeons) who argue for a more cautious approach to the surgery, given the facts that there is no evidence yet of increased survival or prevention of heart attack, that the benefits are temporary and that there are many long-term and short-term risks. These doctors by and large recommend surgery only in the cases of patients with truly disabling angina and severely hampered life-styles who have not been helped by medical therapy even after careful and thorough efforts to control pain with drugs. Surgically conservative physicians argue that new drugs such as Propanolol can be extremely efficient in relieving chest pain if serious efforts are made to treat the symptoms without surgery. These doctors also consider the condition of the left ventricle of the heart, and tend to recommend surgery only when the left ventricle is relatively undamaged, for patients who have congestive heart failure and poor left ventricular function stand a much higher chance of dying in surgery and a lower chance of getting any benefit from the operation. Some conservative physicians are also recommending the surgery for the small percentage of patients (about 10 percent of those with chest pain) who have severe disease of the left main coronary artery, since these patients are very likely to have a heart attack if treated only with medical therapy.

In between these two groups of physicians are those who seem to make judgments for individual patients on an ad hoc rather than a systematic basis, probably basing their decisions on their feelings about individual patients.

Despite the divisions of opinion about the operation it is likely that for a while at least (for reasons I shall discuss later) the trend will be in the direction of doing more surgery.

More individuals with chest pain will be referred for surgical treatment even before careful medical management is attempted and more patients who do not suffer from medically uncontrolled pain will be told to undergo diagnostic tests and thereafter referred to surgery. Some categories of patients now being sent to surgery will be removed from the list of good surgical candidates, for they will be found to be of the types that do better without surgery; their places, however, will be more than filled with other categories of patients who will be recruited more actively than they are at present. As one surgeon remarked, there has rarely been a situation in the history of surgery where surgical specialists find they have less to do rather than more.

WHAT PATIENTS BELIEVE ABOUT THE OPERATION

Patients and the public are generally misled into holding a much more optimistic view of the surgery than facts should allow. Partly they are influenced by media coverage that dramatizes the effectiveness of surgery, for the media typically report spectacular results. Another way patients are misled is through the selective statistics and information they hear from doctors. As many studies show, surgical mortality rates and graft patency vary widely according to the experience of the surgeon and the hospital. Yet it is almost certainly the case that patients are told the most promising statistics. Patients considering the operation are frequently told, for example, that "mortality rates for this operation have now been brought below two percent" even though their actual chances of dying in surgery may be much higher according to their particular condition and where they are having the operation. Many surgeons resent some of the hospitals that boast the lowest mortality rates, because they suspect that these hospitals use looser indications for surgery and operate on relatively healthy patients. Still, even surgeons with higher mortality rates can make use of the attractive figures of their competitors. As one surgeon explained, "Well, even if they make my statistics look bad, they provide a service for all of us because if we can say that it is possible to bring the mortality rate down below one percent then we can persuade a lot more cardiologists to refer their patients to surgery." [28]

Patients are misled not only because they are told the most promising statistics, but also because they are *not* told of the many risks and limitations of the operation. Most patients, then, come to confuse relief with cure, and do not realize that the surgery will provide them with only temporary relief and not stop the natural course of their disease.

Some surgically conservative doctors claim that the pressure to do the operation comes from patients, and that they are unable to discourage surgically oriented patients who want to have something done for their pain. However, it is probably more typical that badly informed patients are influenced by the enthusiasm of physicians. Once a patient is admitted to a hospital for diagnostic tests, he is likely to be carried along the path to operation, and to be left feeling that he needs the operation to save his life. Asked how it is that patients are not fully aware of the risks and limitations of the surgery, one surgeon explained, "Well, you have to help a patient through an operation like this. So we would probably say, 'It's very effective in relieving pain and we have reason to believe it will prolong your life. If I were you, I would have it.' " [29]

Many patients report even stronger encouragement from their doctors. When asked how they made the decision to have the operation, many answer that they see no alternatives if they want to avoid a heart attack. As one patient explained, "The doctor said I really didn't have a choice. That if I didn't have the operation I probably wouldn't be around next Christmas." [30]

Given the fact that there has been so much controversy about this operation within the medical profession, one may wonder why more of this disagreement has not reached the public's attention. Part of the answer is relatively simple. One research cardiologist privately expressed his opinion that 80 percent of bypass operations being done are "worthless" apart from temporarily relieving symptoms, and he added that many well-informed physicians shared his judgment. Asked why none of them had made a public statement he explained that it was a very "sensitive area" in medicine, and that just as the benefits of the operation had not been proven, so had they not been disproven. Most important, he added, was the fact that any doctor who made a strong public statement against the operation was likely to hear a lot of angry responses from other physicians.[31]

II—LACK OF REGULATION IN THE DEVELOPMENT AND APPLICATION OF BYPASS SURGERY

The manner in which coronary bypass surgery developed in the United States reflects the laissez-faire attitudes and structures that characterize American medicine. Two facts are central in this matter. First, there are no restrictions on how experimental surgical procedures can be used in American medicine. Second, although there is some indication that specialists within surgery may soon try to exclude less specialized general surgeons from dipping into their areas of practice, it is generally the case that surgeons loyally support one another in resisting any regulation or restriction on surgical practice.

There is no equivalent of the F.D.A. for surgery. The Food and Drug Administration is supposed to make sure that new drugs and medical therapies are tested and approved before being released for general use. But as its title implies, the Food and Drug Administration has no jurisdiction over surgery or experimental operations.

Thus when coronary bypass surgery was introduced it was done, and continues to be done by any cardiac surgeon, experienced with it or not, who chooses to do it. There has never been any requirement for reporting experiences with it. There is no systematic check on mortality rates. Even in its initial stages it was never restricted to a few centers with experienced surgeons who both had the greatest skill and experience and who could also have kept records of all outcomes in all cases in order to determine the operation's usefulness, limitations, best timing, and appropriate selection of patients. Instead, the operation was quickly adopted for wide clinical use even before it was well understood. There is still no way of knowing exactly who is doing it, for what reasons, and with what results.

As several physicians have pointed out, the lack of control in the application of coronary bypass surgery is not atypical of surgical practice. There are many examples of operations which were widely performed (and some continue to be widely done) which have never been demonstrated by controlled studies to be useful or effective. These include radical mastectomy for stage I cancer, tonsillectomy in many situations, portacaval shunts for esophageal varices, and gastric freezing for peptic ulcer.[1,14] In fact, there has been a particularly disturbing pattern in the history of surgical procedures for coronary artery disease. Earlier operations, now discontinued, included the "poudrage" method of purposely irritating and scarring the heart in order supposedly to encourage the growth of new vessels. More recently, the internal mammary artery ligation procedure was a popular operation performed on patients suffering from coronary disease until it was later shown to be ineffective, and replaced by the contemporary method using vein grafts.[1,6,14] To those who urge a more conservative approach to bypass surgery in light of these past procedures which were enthusiastically endorsed only to be later found useless, one leading surgeon wrote: "Whatever surgical efforts were expended before are of historical interest only, and it does little good to dwell on past failures; besides, the statute of limitations for an earlier era should have expired by now." [32]

In 1969 a committee of leading cardiac surgeons and specialists (the Intersociety Commission for Heart Disease Resources) was convened by various medical and surgical associations to issue guidelines about what resources (for example, equipment, personnel, and minimum case loads) a hospital should have in order to properly undertake heart surgery. The committee made several suggestions about what the "optimal" resources should be for attempting cardiac surgery.[33] But when attempts were later made to use these guidelines to regulate the practice of cardiac surgery, members of the committee protested that they had not intended for their suggestions to be used in a way that would constitute a "restraint of trade." [34] In their original report in 1972 the committee referred to a survey conducted in 1969 which indicated that *of 480 hospitals then doing open heart surgery, only 25 met the guidelines suggested by the committee.* Since the committee's recommendations were suggested guidelines rather than restrictions with any authority, *it is still the case today that most hospitals doing open heart surgery do not meet the guidelines recommended in 1972 or in the updated report.*[17]

One leading cardiac surgeon who had served on the committee was asked why there were no controlled studies of cardiac bypass surgery to determine the parameters of its usefulness before it was widely used, and why all hospitals are allowed to do it, even when they fall far short of the ICHD guidelines. He gave the following reply:

"Well, you could say that we sacrifice people, and some people die, but people are dying off like flies anyway. They're dying from heart attacks in the millions. And you could say that there are too many people anyway."

When asked why there are no regulations to insure that only qualified doctors do the operation, he answered:

"Eventually everything will balance out so that the incompetent doctors get driven out of the market. In coronary surgery you find out when patients die because of incompetence—there are too many people involved for the surgeon's mistakes to go unnoticed. If I were doing a gall bladder operation I could see a patient in my office, decide to do an operation with or without an x-ray, carry out the operation with the help of a nurse, and no one would ever be looking over my shoulder. But in cardiac surgery there are more people involved. With a stomach operation you can go an inch too far in either direction and nothing will happen, but in coronary bypass surgery you can't. It's very exacting and technically demanding and eventually your bad results will become obvious and you won't get any more referrals. It's like choosing a hotel—you come to a city and need a hotel, and at first they all look the same from the outside. So you might go to any one of them. But if you go to a hotel that turns out to be full of cockroaches and there's noise all night, you won't go back to that hotel. It's the same with coronary artery surgery. When doctors see that some surgeons have poor results, they'll stop sending their patients to those doctors. Eventually things will balance out. Rigid controls are no good. We have the best medical care system because it's competitive." [35]

Despite this surgeon's faith that incompetent doctors are driven out of the market, there is considerable evidence (from variations in long-term mortality rates) that incompetent surgical teams *continue* to get referrals and do business because mortality rates are *not* systematically recorded and are certainly *not* distributed as advisory information. Even in cases where observant doctors in the local community stop referring patients, incompetent surgery teams continue to get referrals from out-of-town physicians who are unaware of the poor results. Because hospitals and physician colleagues systematically overlook medical errors and because there are no structures for monitoring incompetence, the only time incompetence gets widely exposed is when there is a public scandal. In addition to this problem, it is also a significant fact that cardiologists have a personal and financial interest in referring patients to surgeons working in their own hospitals, however they may evaluate the surgeons' capabilities.

Surgeons have also resisted the efforts of medical doctors and their organizations to restrict the application of coronary artery surgery. At one meeting of the American Heart Asso-

ciation the sentiment was expressed that surgeons should go
slowly with the operation until the long-term results are in.
In response to that suggestion, one leading cardiac surgeon
replied: "The American Heart Association and its leaders
have a perfect right to their opinion but are not in a position
to influence one way or another this development of events." [36]

As they stressed in their updated report [17] the members of
the ICHD committee emphasized that it had not been their
intention for their guidelines to be used to restrict the practice
of surgery. As some explained in interviews, they were partly
referring to a few incidents in which local insurance organizations had attempted to enforce the guidelines by refusing to
pay hospitals doing heart surgery that did not meet the committee's suggested standards.

One such incident involved the actions of Herbert Denenberg, when he was insurance commissioner of the state of
Pennsylvania. It had been Denenberg's judgment that there
were far too many open heart surgery teams operating in
the state, and since many did not meet the guidelines suggested by the committee, he had attempted to create a Blue
Cross-Blue Shield contract that would eventually phase out
those surgery programs falling short of the guidelines. Part
of his reason was the obvious evidence that hospitals were
financing these unnecessary programs by raising the daily
hospital rates for *all* patients, and by as much as ten dollars
per day.[37] Denenberg was unable to carry out this reform
because of the resistance of the local physicians.

In their updated report (1975) the members of the ICHD
committee emphasized that the purpose of their original report was not to set minimal standards for doing heart surgery.
They prefaced their new report with this qualification, even
though they conceded that a serious problem still exists with
regard to the proliferation of cardiac surgery programs:

> Within the past three decades cardiac surgical teams have been
> organized throughout the United States. Some have failed be-
> cause of poor planning, inadequate staff and lack of material
> resources. Others have had case loads so marginal as to raise

serious questions about their effectiveness, safety and economic soundness. Even today the majority of cardiac surgery programs appear to be operating well below capacity. . . . With the increase in patients attendant on the introduction of direct coronary artery surgery, many hospitals are again being stimulated to expand their programs to meet an apparent or actual need, sometimes under the mistaken impression that patients undergoing coronary artery surgery do not require the same depth of staff capability, preoperative evaluation, postoperative management and systematic follow-up as do traditional cardiac surgery patients. We may, therefore, see once more a proliferation of poorly conceived and poorly planned units with costly duplication of facilities and less-than-optimal care.[17]

Although the committee had urged and continued to maintain that an adequate program should do at least 200 procedures annually, they reported their most recent figures (1971) indicating that of all 470 hospitals doing open heart surgery, 9.6 percent were doing only 1–9 cases per year, 19.8 percent were doing 10–49, 23.4 percent were doing 50–99 cases, 22.3 percent were doing 100–199, and *only 14.9 percent were doing over 200 cases per year,* the number they had suggested three years before as an optimal case load. Although there had been some improvement over the 3.1 percent that had met the standard in 1961,[17] it is uncertain whether the tremendous expansion of coronary artery surgery and its facilities has worsened or improved the picture since 1971.

The overexpansion of hospitals and cardiac programs has by now become a widely acknowledged problem in medicine, and some attempts (in New York City and in California) have been made to restrict further expansion until a hospital can demonstrate a need for a new cardiac surgery program in its community. Although regulation is certainly needed, attempts to deal with the problem through piecemeal actions will probably not be successful, as the following situation illustrates:

An administrator of one community hospital in California explained that his hospital was under some pressure to open a new cardiac surgery program because of a new state restriction supposedly aimed at reducing unneeded and dangerous programs. The California Licensing Act of 1975 specified that neither cardiac catheterization laboratories nor open heart surgery programs would be allowed in any hospitals that did not have both facilities. The reasoning behind the restriction was to centralize programs and to ensure patient safety. In a small number of cases, an emergency arises during a catheterization (a technique for studying the heart) which requires immediate surgery (and thus open-heart surgery facilities) for the patient. In the case of this particular hospital, the administrator was not particularly anxious to invest in a new cardiac surgery program, especially because his hospital was very close to a major center for cardiac surgery. He maintained that in the case of an emergency he could get a patient over into the operating room of the nearby medical center in just ten minutes and perhaps in less time than surgery could be arranged for a patient within the medical center itself. But, as he explained, his hospital had already invested several hundred thousand dollars in equipment for its catheterization laboratory and they could not afford to lose that investment. So he was now preparing to invest another hundred thousand dollars to finance a new, small cardiac surgery program. He reported that his case was not unusual, and that many hospitals in California were preparing to do the same thing.[38]

This case illustrates how an isolated attempt to restrict programs in the cause of safety and economy may itself create the opposite effect.

What has been the result of this lack of control in the development of coronary bypass surgery? Since many of the facts about the operation are still unknown, it is hard to answer this question fully, but some disturbing facts are already clear. Because the operation was widely applied before its risks and limitations were known, many early patients were "sacrificed" in the sense that their conditions were later shown to be the kind *not* well suited to surgery. To be more precise, severe congestive heart failure, poor left ventricular function, immediate myocardial infarction and single vessel disease are among the conditions now widely felt to be *contraindications* of surgery, but many patients in these categories underwent the operation in the early days, sometimes with disastrous results. For example, one researcher pointed out that patients who had severe preoperative heart failure were likely to have neither symptomatic nor objective improvement after surgery. Furthermore, these patients have a very high surgical mortality risk: One group reported a 37 percent mortality rate one year after operation with such patients, with relief of symptoms in only 20 percent.[26]

It might be argued that the first patients receiving an experimental operation are always "sacrificed" since the limitations and dangers are learned only after the surgery has been tried for a while. But if surgical innovations were subjected to more careful practice and reporting, it would seem that important information would be yielded more quickly.

The lack of control in coronary bypass surgery has other obvious ill effects. It has been demonstrated that the proliferation of unneeded cardiac surgery teams creates not only unnecessary public expense but a situation in which badly equipped and inexperienced surgeons are doing operations under a competitive pressure to find more cases in order to keep their programs alive—a situation likely to lead to questionable judgment in many situations.

It is not surprising that where there is an incentive to find surgical cases, the indications for surgery become looser. Thus many physicians have informally observed (but without wishing to be quoted) that in areas of the country with large numbers of private community hospitals and a high concentration of cardiac surgeons, bypass operations are more likely to be performed with questionable indications.

Similarly, in prepaid health plans where it would be financially disadvantageous for doctors to recommend bypass surgery (as well as where such surgery conflicts with institutional philosophy) there seems to be a remarkably lower rate of decisions to operate compared with such decisions made by doctors paid by fee-for-service. This is the case even though the patient populations in the two situations are similar and likely to have comparable symptoms. And, expectedly, there has been little enthusiasm for bypass surgery in countries with a much smaller ratio of thoracic surgeons to population. The United States has a ratio of thoracic surgeons many times greater than any other nation. All of these facts suggest that what is seen as an "indication" for surgery is not based merely or primarily upon scientific evidence but also on the basis of the financial incentives of those who make the judgments. Under such circumstances, the dangers of proliferating cardiac surgery programs becomes all the more obvious.

What is the solution to the problem of lack of regulation in surgery? Some physicians have argued that there is a "double standard" and that surgical practice is not subjected to the same external control as is medical practice, and that it should be.[15] One physician who is critical of bypass surgery made the following argument in 1971 (the cost of the surgery has doubled or tripled by now):

> Surgical procedures, like drugs, are therapeutic agents. They are introduced to improve the health of man and not to injure him. Saphenous vein grafts for coronary arterial diseases have an operative mortality rate of about 10 percent, a morbidity rate of about 25 percent or more (pulmonary embolism, pericarditis, pneumonia, pleuritis, hemorrhage, myocardial infarction, cardiac causalgia, and many other complications and disturbances in health), associated pain and suffering of 100 percent, and a cost of $3,000 to $6,000 or more to the patient. The grafts do not cure the coronary arterial disease, about 25 percent of the shunts close within 2 years, and the surgical procedure has never been subjected to any control studies such as sham operation or "double-blind" evaluation.
>
> Imagine any capable cardiologist prescribing a pill that had never been subjected to double-blind control studies, that might kill 1 out of 10 patients, hurt 25 percent, produce pain and suffering in 100 percent, cost $3,000 to $6,000 to the patient, and

never cure him! Not only would the cardiologist not prescribe such a pill, but also the F.D.A. would not allow the pill to reach the market and the public.[39]

Indeed, there is beginning to be some call among medical physicians for an equivalent of the F.D.A. for surgery. Some doctors feel that if new medical therapies have to be tested through controlled randomized studies before they are released for general use, the same rules should apply to surgical innovations. Medical doctors resent the "double standard."

Cardiac surgeons have frequently argued, on the other hand, that while controlled studies are feasible in medicine (say, with the use of an experimental drug and a placebo) they are impossible in surgery because a patient who wants to have an operation would not be satisfied if he were assigned to a medical control group. It is argued that such a patient would probably "defect" from the study and go to another hospital and another surgeon. Others have complained that it is "unethical" to withhold a treatment one believes to be beneficial just to prove its scientific usefulness, and many surgeons argue that they could not ethically withhold surgery from patients with chest pain. Those who have advocated controlled studies point out, however, that it is unethical *not* to do these studies.[15]

Furthermore, ethical concerns are often difficult to separate from practical ones. Although surgeons have argued that controlled studies are impossible in coronary bypass surgery, they *have* been underway for some time in Veterans Administration hospitals because these patients are not in a position to choose or "defect" from the study, even if they are not assigned to the form of treatment they prefer. This suggests that some of the resistance to controlled studies of surgery emerges at least partially from concern with losing patients to another doctor rather than solely from ethical concerns.

The resistance to regulation is of course part of the entire laissez-faire structure of American surgery. Requirements for randomized control studies before approving surgical procedures are often more easily tolerated in countries with socialized medicine. And interestingly, coronary bypass surgery had not been approved for wide use in Great Britain at the time of a recent report.[1]

Finally, surgeons often protest that there are more unique factors in each surgical case, as opposed to medical treatments, and that these make it impossible to make generalizations or keep records needed for controlled studies. In answer to this argument, some physicians point out that surgeons *could* record all the information that is needed for scientific evaluation *if* they were willing to spend the extra half hour that it would take in each case. It is also suggested that surgeons are more "individualistic" than medical doctors, and more likely to regard their work as a kind of artistic performance not well suited to scientific evaluation.

Surely some effective regulation is needed. But even if a "surgical F.D.A." were created to evaluate experimental procedures, there is some question about whether it would be very effective in protecting consumers' interests. Considering the power and influence of drug companies over American medicine, it is not surprising that the performance of the F.D.A. has been disappointing, and there is little reason to expect that a surgical F.D.A. would be very different. Quite simply, the same powerful interests that dominate surgical practice are also likely to dominate a committee set up to regulate that practice. Even if fair, controlled studies were required to evaluate surgical innovations, it is not clear what impact those studies would have.

As one researcher has pointed out,[40] even after controlled studies have revealed that particular drugs are ineffective and highly dangerous, physicians continue to prescribe them. A recent dramatic example is the use of oral hypoglycemic drugs for patients with late-onset diabetes. Although several studies (as long as seven years ago) showed that this drug created a substantially higher risk of cardiovascular disease and that large numbers of people taking the drug did not need it, doctors' prescription of the drug continued to increase. In 1973, over 1.4 million Americans were still being treated with the drug.[1, 40]

Although better regulation of surgical experimentation and practice is surely needed, it would be naive to expect that effective regulation in the public interest can easily take place in the context of a multi-billion-dollar industry. Questionable medical practice is not just the result of mistakes, occasional incompetence, and faulty regulation, but is the outcome of vested interests. An examination of these interests is therefore essential for understanding how particular medical practices, such as coronary bypass surgery, are promoted.

III—WHO PAYS, WHO PROFITS?

In understanding and evaluating the dramatic proliferation of coronary artery surgery it is finally important to consider the interests of each group in the situation, and certain background economic and political factors. It is clear that given: 1) the prevalence of coronary artery disease in our society, 2) the lack of preventive programs, 3) the anxiety-provoking attention heart disease gets in the media and 4) the misleading information given to the public about surgery, that there will be a huge demand for this operation.

Such a demand fits very nicely with the needs of thoracic (chest) surgeons as well. Only a few years ago, before bypass surgery made its impact, the yearly presidential addresses to organizations of thoracic surgeons were pleas for the group to restrict its production of new members.[41, 42, 43] It was felt that there were too many surgeons coming out of the training programs and not enough business for them. Furthermore, it was frequently pointed out that the sources of much of their business were disappearing. Antibiotics were now controlling rheumatic fever leading to heart disease and also pulmonary infections; there was a sharp decrease of advanced pulmonary tuberculosis; there was a declining birth rate; legal sanctions to abort pregnancies of women with rubella and other conditions predisposing to fetal abnormalities had controlled the incidence of congenital diseases, and the anti-smoking campaign is viewed as likely to have some impact as well.[43] Suddenly there seemed to be a crisis in the overproduction of thoracic (including cardiac) surgeons. But in the explosion of coronary artery surgery, the thoracic surgeons have found a new and unlimited source of patients, a source better than anything they have ever had before. As the noted surgeon Francis Moore pointed out in an introduction to a textbook on cardiac surgery, coronary artery disease provides unlimited opportunities for surgeons:

> The future of coronary artery surgery is especially interesting because of its population. Congenital malformations of the heart and advanced valvular disease involve limited statistical fractions of the population. These are defined groups that can be cared for in toto. A "static group" undergoes repair, after which only those cases newly appearing each year become subject to the need for repair. Several of these disease entities are disappearing. In other instances they are of extreme rarity.
>
> By contrast, surgery for coronary artery disease (either by direct, anastomotic, or transplant procedures) involves no such delimited population. In this country and in Western Europe coronary artery disease may be important in as many as 30 percent of the male population reaching the age of 55. In each individual patient the disease is dynamic, changing and evolving from year to year. The potential need for cardiac surgery and its populational potential are very impressive.[44]

The tremendous financial opportunities of bypass surgery for thoracic surgeons are obvious, and need no further comment. But what about for other physicians? Cardiologists (medical heart specialists) who perform preoperative and postoperative procedures are paid much more money for their time and effort than they are paid to manage patients with nonsurgical therapies. Many physicians have observed that the structure of third-party insurance payments predisposes doctors to select treatments involving surgery or expensive diagnostic procedures involving fancy machinery because these earn higher fees and require less doctor time. But even family physicians who do not stand to gain financially by referring patients to cardiologists and surgeons have participated in the trend because they have been frustrated in not knowing what to do for a patient with persistent chest pain.

One may wonder why large numbers of community hospitals are rushing to start cardiac surgery programs at a considerable expense when the vast majority of these facilities are actually underused and constitute a drain on hospital funds.[1, 17, 33]

Part of the answer is that hospitals have seriously overexpanded [45] beyond market need and they are competing with one another for patients and doctors to fill up empty beds. Many hospital directors feel they need the prestige and equipment of cardiac surgery programs in order to attract doctors and their patients. They figure that with a sufficient case load, cardiac surgery can be very lucrative for their hospitals. Furthermore, if national health insurance legislation with an emphasis on payment for "catastrophic illness" rather than other kinds of routine care is passed, and this is likely to happen, there will be even further incentive to invest in programs such as cardiac surgery. In such a case, the federal government would be supporting medical practices involving expensive equipment yielding large profits to large corporations, a not unsurprising development. Eventually the costs of high-technology treatments will become so huge that the government will *have* to restrict these developments by requiring centralized, regional health-care facilities and by restricting the training and production of medical specialists in favor of primary-care physicians who are less likely to use expensive equipment and therapies.

But so far it has been relatively easy for hospitals to expand their facilities beyond the market demand, because of the structure of financing this expansion. Hospitals have been able to obtain funds for uncontrolled capital expansion through direct government subsidies, capital depreciation payments, and "plus" or "surplus" payments over cost of care from Blue Cross, Medicare and Medicaid. All of this money for expanded facilities is contributed by the public, either in the form of direct federal taxes or from increased insurance rates and hospital charges.

Since hospitals have to compete with one another for patients, and since the funds for expansion have been readily available and can be passed off to consumers, the potential for proliferation of high-technology programs like cardiac surgery is immense.

Who is profiting from this explosion of facilities besides doctors and hospital directors? A look at health care costs is illuminating. The total annual expenditures on health care in the United States rose dramatically from 26 billion dollars in 1960 to 67 billion dollars in 1970.[46] And by 1975 American health care cost 118.5 billion dollars, 40 percent of it paid by public funds via federal, state and local governments.[47] The expenditures and the percentage taken from public funds continue to rise rapidly. Many of the same giant corporations that dominate other segments of American industry are also heavily involved in health care.[4,48] Of special interest to coronary bypass surgery and its recent growth is the fact that it is the same electronics industry that suffered some depression after cutbacks in military and defense spending that is now producing expensive diagnostic and monitoring equipment used in heart surgery and in coronary care units. Industries profiting from war and defense are now profiting from health care. Indeed, most of the equipment used in cardiac surgery was originally developed in the space program. It is not surprising that electronics industries would diversify into health care, for hospitals provide a vast market for new applications of the same basic equipment these corporations developed for national military defense. These industries constantly require new large markets for the absorption of their surplus products. Furthermore, as the federal government increasingly finances the cost of health care, it is in a better position to support the development of high-technology medical practices (and thus these industries) by such arrangements as insurance for "catastrophic" illness (rather than for routine health care) and by various kinds of subsidies and research and development grants. The giant corporations can therefore enjoy the same benefits of monopoly and government subsidy in health care they earlier enjoyed in their defense contracts. Nonetheless, the government will soon face a crisis of how it can finance expensive, high-technology treatments for large portions of the population. We may soon observe a contradiction between the government support of medical-technological industries on the one hand and an urgent need to control the costs of health care on the other.

But at the present time, thousands of hospitals, all in competition with each other, will steadily need the increasingly expensive technological equipment which will become obsolete every five years and in need of replacement. Like diseased coronary arteries and surgery, there will be a dynamic "need" for medical technology.

It is usually assumed by the public and even by physicians that this expensive medical technology is beneficial to patients. But such an assumption should not be made. For example, although very expensive coronary care units (involving much of the same equipment used in cardiac surgery) have proliferated across the nation, there is beginning to be some serious doubt about whether these units actually help patients.[49] Characteristically, these costly units were allowed to proliferate before their benefits were carefully evaluated, and like bypass surgery, once this unregulated expansion was put into motion it was more difficult to evaluate or control the innovation.

The unregulated and disturbing expansion of coronary artery bypass surgery should therefore not be seen as an isolated event, or simply the result of insufficiently regulated physicians. It is a part of a current trend in American health care: a pattern of an "engineering" rather than a preventive approach to disease, and a trend toward treatments using expensive technology yielding large profits to giant corporations. These therapies increasingly involve spending a great deal of public money on selected (and usually affluent) patients, at the expense of basic health care for large portions of the population. But ironically, as the case of bypass surgery indicates, it is not clear that even the privileged recipients of these treatments are getting good medical care. Even one enthusiastic cardiac surgeon notes the drawbacks of medical technology:

> This whole gamut of therapy for surgical disease, from heart replacement, replacement of parts, assisted circulation as a holding action, and counterpulsation as a definitive therapy to counterpulsation as a prophylactic measure, will have extended use through improved automation of monitoring and therapeutic devices. Such automation has already proved useful, but it is not without hazards. The complicated but life-saving science fiction world of Intensive Care Units has produced a series of diseases of and in itself. There have been *psychologic* disadvantages including fear, insomnia and the disturbance of diurnal and circadian rhythms. There have been *mechanical* disadvantages stemming from the improper use of respirators, endotracheal tubes and other equipment. There have been *electrical* hazards varying from simple arrhythmias to burns and electrocution while utilizing otherwise life-saving equipment. There have been *chemical* and bacteriologic or *infectious* accidents due to inappropriate patient segregation or incomplete device precautions in the Intensive Care and Coronary Care Units. Finally, *human factors* have included errors in maintenance, use, interpretation and trauma. This new breed of diseases can hardly be called iatrogenic for they are not primarily caused by the doctor. They are not nosocomial or those caused by the house. They are caused by the things immediately about the patient, so for this new disease form a new word has been created: *periontogenic* diseases. Periontogenic describes those diseases the *"genesis"* of which are in "the things about." These diseases will be corrected when they are recognized only to be replaced by new periontogenic diseases as new monitoring and therapeutic equipment is devised.[50]

CONCLUSION

It is unlikely that the growth of technology in medicine, some of it of doubtful benefit, will be stopped in the short run, although the government will eventually face a cost-crisis.

Increasingly, more expensive diagnostic and treatment equipment will be developed. There have recently been suggestions [51] of "medical nemesis" and proposals that we should abandon all of this equipment and return to self-care and a simpler life. But this proposal, while it justifiably cites the irrationality (from the standpoint of benefit to patients) of much of the technology, does not adequately consider *why* health care is turning in these directions. Similarly, arguments that there should be a federal regulatory agency for surgery are important, but they do not take into account the problem that the same groups and interests that heavily influence surgical practice also influence the government and its regulatory agencies, thus making truly public-interested regulation a remote prospect. American medicine is a multi-billion-dollar business. As long as it is the source of huge corporate profits, medical practice and its regulation will be shaped by political and economic considerations as much as by "scientific" ones. What seems like senseless investment in questionable technological devices may become more understandable in the context of these broader economic and social factors.

There has recently been much talk of "necessary" and "unnecessary" surgery. Given the impact of technology on medicine, and the large and growing proportion of health care financed with government (public) funds, it seems appropriate to examine what we mean by "necessary" and "unnecessary." "Necessary" has traditionally been defined in terms of the individual. It has commonly been assumed that a doctor should do everything he or she can for individual patients. But since we have only a finite amount of resources to spend on health care, what is "necessary" or "unnecessary" surgery must be publicly decided and viewed in terms of what best serves the entire society as well as what serves individuals.

Properly placed in a social context, the question of whether coronary artery surgery is "necessary" becomes a more complex matter, and one which should be decided by the public rather than by individual patients and doctors. First of all, it is highly questionable whether the coronary bypass operation is beneficial in the long run to all or most of the people who are having it. It *is* clear that many patients who have had the operation should not have had it, or are unlikely to benefit from it. More careful testing at the beginning before the operation was given widespread application might have saved many patients from surgery we would consider "unnecessary" even by traditional definition. More careful regulation of who may perform the operation and under what indications and circumstances might also eliminate some questionable practice of the surgery.

In the larger context that billions of dollars are being spent on a temporary, palliative procedure for a progressive and chronic disease when correspondingly little is spent on the broader health problems of the nation (including widespread malnutrition and diseases that can be easily and inexpensively prevented and cured), the problem takes on another dimension. We must think of what is necessary for the public good as well as what is necessary for some individuals.

And finally, if our health care system is to truly serve the interests of all Americans instead of the small portion of the population that owns and profits from the industry, it should seem obvious that vast private profits should not be allowed in health care.

NOTES

1. H. Hiatt, "Protecting the Medical Commons: Who Is Responsible?" *New England Journal of Medicine* 293 (1975):235–241.
2. "Does the U.S. Need 80,000 Coronary Angiograms a Day?" *Medical World News* 15, no. 34 (1974):14–16.
3. F. D. Moore, foreword, in John C. Norman, ed., *Cardiac Surgery* (New York: Appleton-Century-Crofts, xiii, 1972).
4. E. A. Krause, "Health and the Politics of Technology," *Inquiry* 8, no. 3 (1971):51–59.
5. E. D. Mundth, "Surgical Measures for Coronary Heart Disease," Part 1, *New England Journal of Medicine* 293, no. 1 (1975): 13–20.
6. R. S. Ross, "Surgery for Coronary Artery Disease Placed in Perspective," *Bulletin of the New York Academy of Medicine* 48, no. 9 (1972):1163–1178.

7. J. M. McNeer et al., "The Nature of Treatment Selection in Coronary Artery Disease," *Circulation* 49 (1974): 606–614.

8. L. A. Cobb, et al., "An Evaluation of Internal Mammary Artery Ligation by Double-Blind Technique," *New England Journal of Medicine* 260 (1959): 1115–1118.

9. E. G. Dimond et al., "Comparison of Internal Mammary Artery Ligation and Sham Operation for Angina Pectoris," *American Journal of Cardiology* 5 (1960):483–486.

10. L. Griffith et al., "Changes in Intrinsic Coronary Circulation and Segmental Ventricular Motion after Saphenous-vein Coronary Bypass Graft Selection," *New England Journal of Medicine* 288, no. 12 (1973):589–595.

11. D. B. Effler, "Myocardial Revascularization," *Chest* 63, no. 1 (1973):79–80.

12. W. S. Aranow and E. A. Stemmer, "Two-Year Follow-Up of Angina Pectoris: Medical or Surgical Therapy," *Annals of Internal Medicine* 82 (1975):208–218.

13. J. M. McNeer et al., "The Nature of Treatment Selection in Coronary Artery Disease," *Circulation* 49 (1974):606–614.

14. T. C. Chalmers, "Randomization and Coronary Artery Surgery," *Annals of Thoracic Surgery* 14 (1972):323–327.

15. D. H. Spodick, "Revascularization of the Heart-Numerators in Search of Denominators," *American Heart Journal* 81, no. 2 (1971):149–157. See also D. H. Spodick, "Aortocoronary Bypass," *Chest* 63, no. 1 (1973):80–81, and D. H. Spodick, "The Surgical Mystique and the Double Standard," *American Heart Journal* 85 (1973):579.

16. E. D. Mundth, "Surgical Measures for Coronary Heart Disease," Part 3, *New England Journal of Medicine* 293, no. 3 (1975):124–130.

17. "Optimal Resources for Cardiac Surgery: Guidelines for Program Planning and Evaluation," Report of the Intersociety Commission for Heart Disease Resources, *Circulation* 52 (1975): A23–37.

18. P. T. Tecklenberg et al., "Changes in Survival and Symptom Relief in a Longitudinal Study of Patients after Bypass Surgery," *Circulation*, Supplement I, 51–52 (1975):I98–104.

19. D. C. Harrison, "The Status of Coronary Bypass Surgery—1975," unpublished paper.

20. B. L. Segal et al., "Saphenous Vein Bypass Surgery for Coronary Artery Disease," *American Journal of Cardiology* 32 (1973): 1010–1013.

21. I. J. Schatz, "The Need to Know," *Chest* 63, no. 1 (1973):82–83.

22. E. D. Mundth, "Surgical Measures for Coronary Heart Disease," Part 2, *New England Journal of Medicine* 293, no. 2 (1975):75–80.

23. D. Brewer et al., "Myocardial Infarction as a Complication of Coronary Bypass Surgery," *Circulation* 47 (1973):58–64.

24. H. Hultgren et al., "Ischemic Myocardial Injury During Coronary Artery Surgery," *American Heart Journal* 82 (1971):624–631.
25. H. Hultgren et al., "Evaluation of Surgery in Angina Pectoris," *American Journal of Medicine* 56 (1974):1–3.
26. E. L. Alderman et al. "Results of Direct Coronary-Artery Surgery for the Treatment of Angina Pectoris," *New England Journal of Medicine* 288, no. 11 (1973):535–539.
27. F. C. Spencer et al., "The Long-Term Influence of Coronary Bypass Grafts on Myocardial Infarction and Survival," *Annals of Surgery* 180, no. 4 (1974):439–451.
28. Anonymous. I interviewed several physicians who are well known in the medical community for either their work or writing on coronary bypass surgery. I conducted the interviews with the understanding that I would not identify individuals or use their names in quotations. Later references marked "Anonymous" refer to these interviews.
29. Anonymous. Research interview.
30. M. Millman, Notes from research on patients' experiences with cardiac surgery.
31. Anonymous. Research interview.
32. D. B. Effler, "Myocardial Revascularization at the Community Hospital Level," *American Journal of Cardiology* 32 (1973):240.
33. "Optimal Resources for Cardiac Surgery," Report of the Intersociety Commission for Heart Disease Resources, *Circulation* 44 (1971):A–221.
34. Anonymous. Research interviews. Also see "Optimal Resources for Cardiac Surgery," Report of the Intersociety Commission for Heart Disease Resources, *Circulation* 52 (1975):A–23.
35. Anonymous. Research interview.
36. "Five Surgeons Reject Criticism of Procedure by AHA," *Medical Tribune*, February 2, 1972.
37. This information was gathered in research interviews.
38. Anonymous. Research interview.
39. G. E. Burch, "Coronary Artery Surgery—Saphenous Vein Bypass," *American Heart Journal* 82, no. 1 (1971):137.
40. T. C. Chalmers, "The Impact of Controlled Trials on the Practice of Medicine," *Mount Sinai Journal of Medicine* 41, no. 6 (1974):753–759.
41. H. Sloan, "The Breeding and Feeding of Thoracic Surgeons," *Annals of Thoracic Surgery* 20, no. 4 (1975):371–385, p. xiii.
42. L. A. Brewer, "A Heritage and a Challenge," *Journal of Thoracic and Cardiovascular Surgery* 68 (1974):177.
43. B. B. Roe, "Whither in Maturity?" *Annals of Thoracic Surgery* 15 (1973):553.
44. F. D. Moore, foreword, in John C. Norman, ed., *Cardiac Surgery* (New York: Appleton-Century-Crofts, 1972) p. xiii.
45. D. Feshbach, "The Dynamics of Hospital Expansion," *Health/ PAC Bulletin* 64 (1975):1–20.

46. R. Alford, "The Political Economy of Health Care: Dynamics Without Change," *Politics and Society* 2 (1972):138.
47. *San Francisco Chronicle*, April 26, 1976, p. 1.
48. S. Kelman, "Toward the Political Economy of Medical Care," *Inquiry* 8, no. 3 (1971):30–38. Also see V. Navarro, "Social Policy Issues: An Explanation of the Composition, Nature, and Functions of the Present Health Sector of the United States," *Bulletin of the New York Academy of Medicine* 51, no. 1 (1975):199–234.
49. H. Waitzkin and J. Fisher, unpublished working paper; and J. Powles, "On the Limitations of Modern Medicine," *Science, Medicine and Man* 1 (1973):1–30.
50. D. E. Harken, "The Future of Cardiac Surgery," in John C. Norman, ed., *Cardiac Surgery* (New York: Appleton-Century-Crofts, 1972) pp. 689–690.
51. I. Illich, *Medical Nemesis* (New York: Pantheon, 1976).